Clinical Skills for Nurses

Second edition

Claire Boyd
RGN, Cert Ed
Practice Development Trainer

WILEY Blackwell

This edition first published 2022

Registered Offices
John Wiley & Sons, Inc., 111 River Street, Hoboken, NJ 07030, USA
John Wiley & Sons Ltd, The Atrium, Southern Gate, Chichester, West Sussex, PO19 8SQ, UK

Editorial Office
9600 Garsington Road, Oxford, OX4 2DQ, UK

For details of our global editorial offices, customer services, and more information about Wiley products visit us at www.wiley.com.

Wiley also publishes its books in a variety of electronic formats and by print-on-demand. Some content that appears in standard print versions of this book may not be available in other formats.

Library of Congress Cataloging-in-Publication Data applied for

PB ISBN: 9781119871545

Cover Design: Wiley
Cover Images: © Rambo182/Getty Images, Chuwy/Getty Images

Set in 9/12pt Trade Gothic LT Std by Straive, Pondicherry, India
Printed and bound by CPI Group (UK) Ltd, Croydon, CR0 4YY

C9781119871545_200622

Contents

Preface

Clinical Skills for Nurses is designed to assist the student healthcare worker in the field of clinical skills. All exercises are related to practice and the healthcare environment, from the acute hospital setting to the community.

The book looks at 16 clinical skills, requested by students like you, and gives a quick, snappy introduction to these skills in a non-threatening manner for you to gain a understanding and as an overview. You can then build on this foundation. For the present you may not be permitted to perform some of the skills, depending on where you are with the training, but that does not stop you from watching them being performed. This will be preparation for the day when you will be expected, often after a formal training event, to undertake them with your own patients.

I talk about 'patients' but the book applies to service users and residents in the community setting as well. The paediatric nurse has not been forgotten, with information given throughout that incorporates this branch of nursing.

The book uses many activities and questions to check your understanding, and is laid out in a simple-to-follow, step-by-step approach. Each chapter ends with a 'test your knowledge' section to relate everything you have learned to your practice. The aim of this book is to start the individual on a journey through many healthcare-related exercises to build confidence and competence; from day one to qualification, and beyond. It has been compiled using quotes and tips from student nurses themselves; it is a book by students for students. I just wish a book like this had been around when I did my nursing training!

Claire Boyd
Bristol
April 2022

Introduction

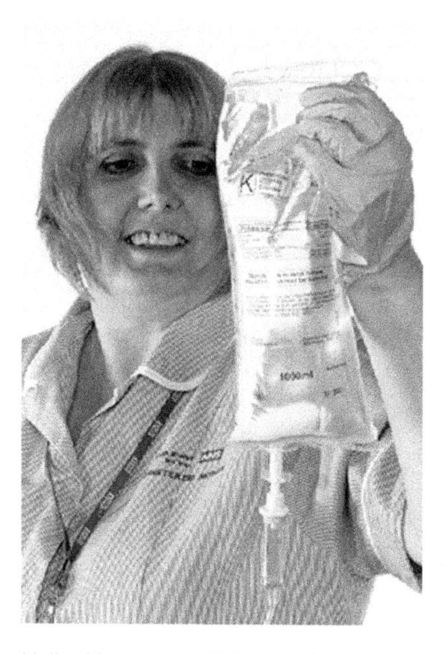

Hello. My name is Claire and I have been a practice development trainer for many years in a large NHS trust training qualified nurses and midwives, student nurses, Assistant Practitioners, Nursing Associates, Physiotherapists, Operating Department Practitioners, Nursing Assistants, Community Carers and even Doctors in clinical skills. I have been a nurse for over 35 years. Yes, that is me above so I hope the picture has not put you off reading this book! Just to note, I wear glasses and had to take them off for the photo as the light reflected on the lens and I could have been holding up a kitten for all I know/could see!

During my career, I will be honest, there have been good days and bad days; good days when I felt I had made a difference to those I had cared for and bad days when a patient died and when I felt I was just 'fire-fighting' during 'winter pressures'. But in all my years of nursing, I have never seen anything quite like the effect of the COVID-19 pandemic within the NHS and the community care setting.

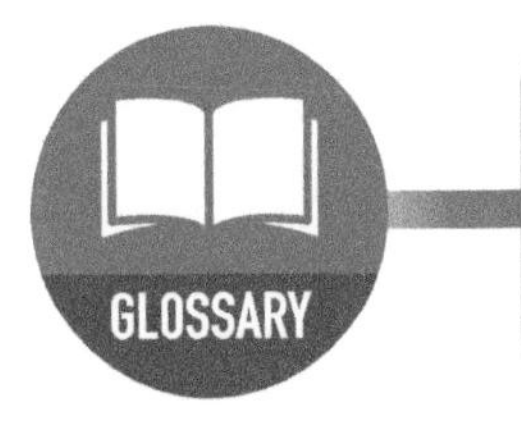

Winter pressures

During the winter period, demand for services tends to increase significantly with the onset of cold weather (e.g. slips, trips, and falls, and the flu virus).

Healthcare staff were physically and emotionally exhausted like never before. Here in the West of England where I live, we had news reports of staff in care homes sleeping in tents in the gardens of the care homes to 'bubble' their care environment and protect their service users and residents, foregoing going home at the end of their shifts to their own families. True care and compassion. Also, hospital staff working extra shifts to cover for their colleagues and working in areas of the hospital that they were not familiar with, helping to 'plug gaps' in care, heaping more pressure on their already intolerable stress and exhaustion levels. Nurses and student healthcare workers suddenly found themselves caring for ventilated patients, the essentials of 'proning', suctioning tracheostomised patients and getting up to speed with clinical skills they did not have or required updating on (e.g. urinary catheterising patients). To say it was difficult times, is putting it mildly!!

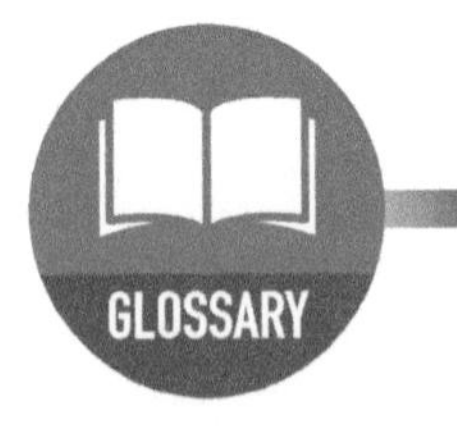

Proning

Proning is the process of lying a patient stomach/face down to boost blood oxygen saturation levels.

This book is designed to assist your practice and is designed for all healthcare students (and qualified nurses, if your skills are rusty, overseas nurses and those returning to practice). This is the second edition of this book and the ethos of the series remains 'for nurses, by nurses' as it is the carers who have informed me what they wanted included in the book. With that in mind, I have been asked to include the following in this second edition of the book:

- information added about aseptic non-touch technique – tick
- information on NEWS 2 – tick

- information added about moisture lesions – tick
- information added about constipation – tick
- information regarding the PureWick female external catheter (students had seen this device on their clinical placements) – tick
- pointers to websites – tick
- more 'test your knowledge' questions – tick and double tick!

I was also informed that they felt four of the skills from the *Care Skills for Nurses* book in the series would be better placed in this clinical skills book, namely:

- continence care – tick
- stoma care – tick
- performing an electrocardiogram – tick
- anaphylaxis – tick.

All your wishes have been incorporated, as requested, in this new edition. Hence this book now looks at 16 clinical skills as opposed to the last edition of 12.

Reading the skills in this book will give you the underpinning knowledge of how the skill should be performed, which you can then build on. It is designed to be small enough to be transportable (in work bags, should you wish for reference). However, it does not make you competent to undertake the skill: You will need to liaise with your university, placement area (hospital or community setting policies), mentor and so on, as to the skills you can perform, as many of these skills require teaching and competency assessment. Performing the skills is also dependent on where you are with your training. For example, a first-year student nurse will be unable to perform the clinical skill of male catheterisation, even under supervision, until they have qualified and most likely also attended a training session.

Throughout you will find Glossary boxes (as above) and as always tips and hints by students, just like you, throughout the book.

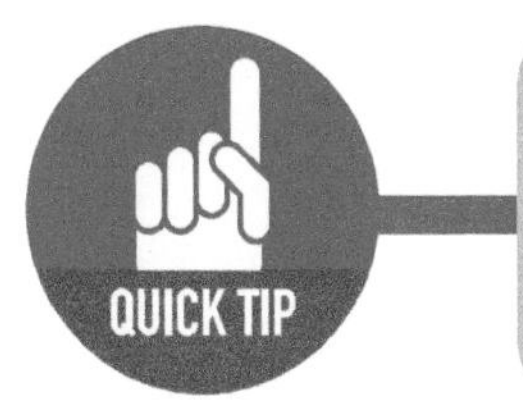

Even if you don't feel confident in performing a skill, don't relay this to the patient as it does not instil confidence in them!

I hope that I have made the writing style informal but brief, as though I am sitting beside you in your clinical placement. All the answers to the activities, questions and 'test your knowledge' exercises can be found at the back of the book.

Acknowledgements

First thanks go to the many wonderful healthcare students I have taught in clinical skills. Believe me when I say that learning has been a two-way process. Again, as in other books in the Student Survival Skills series, it is their tips and quotes that have made this book what it is.

Acknowledgements also go to North Bristol NHS Trust and all my friends and colleagues in the Staff Development Department.

Thanks also go to Tom Marriott at Wiley and to Magenta Styles for first approaching me to begin this series of books. Thanks also to Jane Moody for editorial services and Anne Hunt (Managing Editor) and Adalfin Jayasingh (Content Refinement Specialist).

Special thanks also to BD Diagnostics and Serious Hazards of Blood Transfusion (SHOT) for allowing reproduction of information and diagrams.

This book is dedicated to my loving family: my husband Rob (for the photographs), Simon, Louise and David, and my two wonderful grandsons, Owen and Rhys.

Chapter 1

ASEPTIC NON-TOUCH TECHNIQUE AND INFECTION PREVENTION

Clinical Skills for Nurses, Second Edition. Claire Boyd.

LEARNING OUTCOMES

By the end of this chapter you will have an understanding of the aseptic non-touch technique (ANTT) and be able to define it. You will also be able to describe the ANTT framework, list the ANTT principles and be able to apply ANTT to your practice.

Performing any clinical skills we must first consider infection control principles to reduce incidences of healthcare acquired infections (HCAIs) and community acquired infections. We first need to refresh our understanding of some of these micro-organisms. Table 1.1 shows just four of the micro-organism culprits.

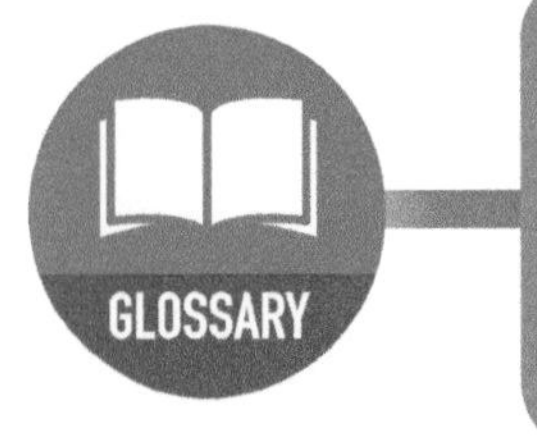

Healthcare acquired infection (HCAI)

Also known as healthcare associated infections. These are infections that people get while they are receiving healthcare for another condition. HCAIs are a significant cause of illness and death and they can have serious emotional, financial and medical consequences.

Table 1.1 Four types of micro-organisms.

Micro-organism	Examples
Bacteria: Gram positive	*Clostridium difficile*, staphylococcus
Bacteria: Gram negative	Salmonella, gonorrhoeae
Mycobacteria	Tuberculosis, leprosy
Virus	Herpes zoster: chicken pox, shingles, norovirus, coronavirus
Fungi (superficial)	Thrush, ringworm
Protozoa	Plasmodium (cause of malaria) Cryptosporidium (can cause gastroenteritis)

MICRO-ORGANISMS

Bacteria, viruses, fungi or other less common pathogens can cause HCAIs. The most well-known include those caused by methicillin-resistant *Staphylococcus aureus* (MRSA) and *Clostridium difficile* (C-diff).

Table 1.1 only shows the 'bad' micro-organisms, known as **pathogenic** microbes. But not all bacteria are bad – the 'good' micro-organisms, known as **commensal** microbes, actually live in or on the human body and help the body: vitamin K, which is necessary to regulate our blood clotting processes, is produced by some of these good bacteria.

DID YOU KNOW?

It has been estimated that 1 kg of an adult's total body weight is composed of bacteria, known as microflora, which are beneficial to the human body.

Just one of those good-guy bacteria is known as *Lactobacillus acidophilus*. This bacterium helps us by:

- supporting digestive function
- supporting the health of the immune system
- supporting the health of the urinary tract
- improving vaginal microflora in women
- enhancing absorption of nutrients
- relieving abdominal cramps, gases, and diarrhoea.

Micro-organisms already present in the body only cause problems when the body's defences are weakened (due to ill health) or breached by surgery or other medical procedures. Within the healthcare environment we are generally more concerned about pathogenic micro-organisms.

MIASMA

Since 100 BCE, our ancestors were aware that disease could be spread by 'imperceptible particles' entering the body; In short that the air around us is not pure, and if you were unlucky, this bad air or 'miasma' could cause disease or death if breathed in. Later on, surgeons would have sulphur burnt where they would operate, to purify the air, creating a lovely aroma of rotten eggs! This rudimental understanding of microbes had not yet equated good health with good hand hygiene.

DID YOU KNOW?

The airborne germs we breathe in includes bacteria, fungi, moulds, viruses, and volatile organic compounds, which are chemicals that easily dissolve in water or vaporise into air.

How Are Micro-organisms Spread?

Micro-organisms are not solely spread through the air; The six potential routes are:

- Direct contact, for example kissing or sexual contact
- Indirect contact, for example contaminated hands touching surfaces or other people
- Airborne, for example sneezing or coughing or through disturbance of dust when cleaning
- Faecal–oral, for example not washing hands after going to the toilet and then preparing food and ingesting it
- Animal vector, for example mosquito bite inserting micro-organisms into the body causing malaria
- Bloodborne, for example sharing dirty needles, used equipment or by infected blood products.

Five Moments of Hand Hygiene

As our knowledge about micro-organisms increased, we also became much more aware of the importance in healthcare of correct hand washing. The World Health Organization (2009) developed the five moments of hand hygiene, suggesting when we should wash our hands:

- before patient contact
- before an aseptic task
- after body fluid exposure risk
- after patient contact
- after contact with patient surroundings.

It is all well and good knowing when to wash your hands, but it must be performed correctly.

Correct Hand Washing

A simple but effective means of protecting patients from nosocomial infection is hand washing, which is considered to be the most basic but vital infection control measure. Healthcare practitioners are taught the six-point hand washing technique:

1. Palm to palm.
2. Right palm over left dorsum and left palm over right dorsum.
3. Palm to palm fingers interlocked.
4. Back of fingers to opposing palms with fingers interlocked.
5. Rotational rubbing of right thumb clasped in left palm and vice versa.
6. Rotational rubbing backwards and forwards with clasped fingers at right hand in left palm and vice versa.

The gold standard is to use liquid soap on wet hands and to dry the hands thoroughly.

The Chain of Infection

We now know how micro-organisms are spread and how effective correct hand washing is, but we also need to be aware of the chain of infection. The chain of infection has six links; break one of the links and the spread of infection is prevented. The six links are:

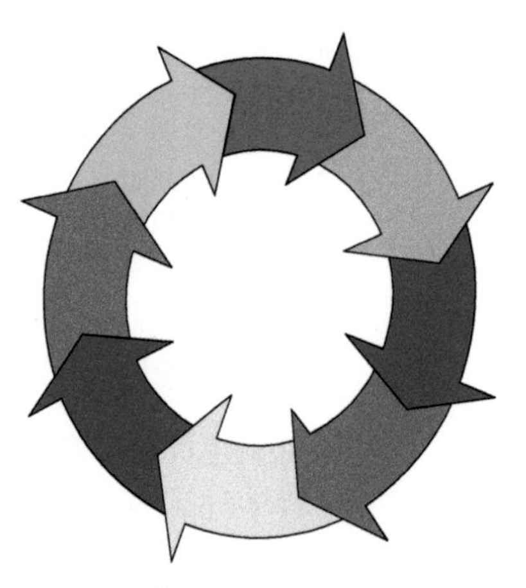

1. An infectious agent, such as MRSA or norovirus.
2. A reservoir, such as people, food, water.
3. A way out of the body, such as, faeces, urine, sneezing.
4. A method of spread, such as contact by hand or equipment, droplets, airborne.
5. A way into the body, such as breaks in the skin, mucous membrane, inhalation.
6. A susceptible host such as elderly individuals or those with poor immune systems (cancer patients, newborn).

Today, healthcare workers are trained in infection control principles and our knowledge has somewhat increased since the miasma theory days! However, we still have much to learn as numbers of patients contracting infections in either the hospital or community setting are far too high. HCAIs pose a serious risk to patients, staff and visitors, and substantial costs to the NHS and care providers, and significant morbidity to those infected. Individuals have the right to expect that they are being safely cared for, with staff trained in infection control principles to minimise their chances of catching an infection.

POOR PRACTICE

As our knowledge in infection control principles have increased, our execution of this knowledge still needs to be addressed.

At the start of my nursing career as a student on placement, I once saw a registered midwife putting on sterile gloves to empty a new mother's urinary catheter bag. Clearly, this healthcare professional had not quite understood the basic principles of infection control, as non-sterile gloves and apron would have sufficed. I have more recently seen a male patient having a urinary catheter inserted with the nurse wearing two pairs of sterile gloves (known as the 'double gloving' technique). We know today that the bottom pair of sterile gloves is *not* sterile because of the pores in the gloves. This practice should no longer be seen when conducting aseptic techniques.

Years ago, it was all very confusing, not least because we would use the term 'sterile technique' and 'aseptic technique' interchangeably. Sterile and aseptic are not the same thing.

DID YOU KNOW?

Double gloving is acceptable practice in surgery/operating theatres as it does provide an additional level of protection against penetration of the gloves by surgical instruments.

What Does It All Mean?

In the healthcare sector, we have known for many years the devastation that the harmful germs can inflict but the terminology we use to describe the technique we are using to reduce contamination has been less clear, if not downright confusing. For example, when performing any dressing change in the ward area, we would wait some time for the dust to settle after bed making and then refer to this dressing change as 'a sterile technique'. In reality, this is totally incorrect, as microbes would still be floating around in the air – just because we can't see them, does not mean that they aren't there!

Note: It is still good practice to wait for some time after bed-making before changing dressings in clinical areas.

It is not possible to achieve a true sterile technique outside the controlled environment of a specially designed operating theatre or sterile cabinet. Table 1.2 shows the definitions of aseptic technique, ANTT, clean and sterile techniques.

A full risk assessment must be conducted to establish which technique is to be employed prior to undertaking the clinical skill.

Note: sterilised equipment can only be considered sterile inside unopened packaging. Once the pack has been opened, it is instantly exposed to airborne organisms and is therefore considered aseptic. The sterile technique employs sterile fields, sterile gowns, masks, sterile gloves, sterile supplies and surgical hand rub.

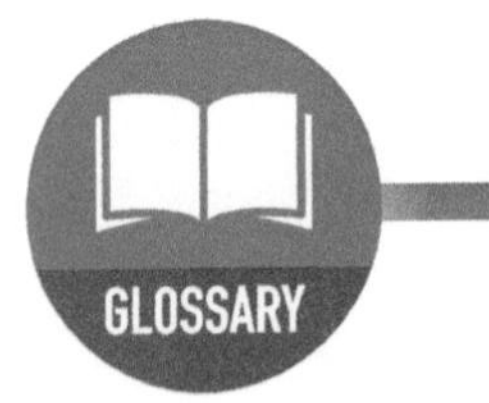

Pathogenic
The ability to cause or produce disease.
Key parts Any part of a piece of equipment used during aseptic technique that will increase the risk of infection if contaminated by infectious material.

Table 1.2 Definitions of aseptic, aseptic non-touch, clean and sterile technique.

Technique	Definition
Aseptic	**'Without organisms'. The principle aim of an aseptic technique is to protect the patient from contamination by pathogenic organisms during medical and nursing procedures.**
Aseptic technique	**Minimising the sterility of a product during handling or preparation. Using this technique is about maintaining the sterility of already sterile objects.**
Aseptic non-touch technique	**Practice of avoiding contamination by not touching key elements, known as 'key parts', such as the tip of a needle or the surface of a sterile dressing where it will be in contact with the wound.**
Clean technique	**A modified aseptic technique that aims to avoid introducing micro-organisms to a susceptible site. The use of sterile equipment is not crucial.**
Sterile technique	**Aims to achieve total freedom from *all* micro-organisms. It is not possible to achieve a true sterile technique outside the controlled environment of a specially designed operating theatre.**

STANDARD AND SURGICAL ASEPTIC NON-TOUCH TECHNIQUE

As we have seen in Table 1.2, a widely used method of aseptic technique is known as ANTT. Performing clinical skills using the ANTT approach is achievable both in the clinical and non-clinical settings such as hospital wards and patients' homes.

There are two types of ANTT, one of which is used in more acute procedures. The two ANTT can be seen in Table 1.3.

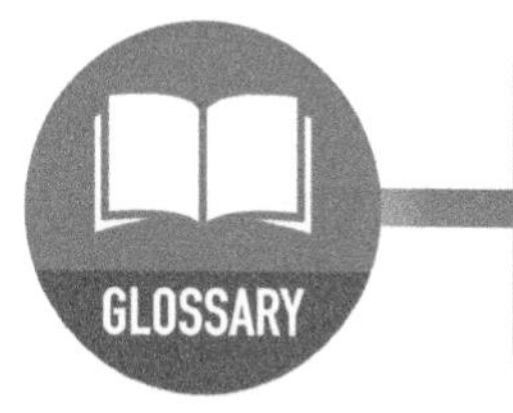

Aseptic field

An aseptic field is a controlled working space that contains and protects procedure equipment from contamination. An aseptic field must be prepared immediately prior to use and not left unattended.

Table 1.3 Standard and surgical aseptic non-touch technique.

	Standard	Surgical
Technique	Technically simple, using non-sterile gloves Employs general aseptic field used for carrying out procedure Short duration	Technically complex, performed using sterile gloves and in operating theatres, usually involving extended time frame
Use	Procedures such as inserting peripheral cannulas, venepuncture, taking blood cultures, intravenous therapy, respiratory suctioning	Procedures involving large open sites Only sterilised equipment can be placed on a critical aseptic field

PRINCIPLES OF ASEPTIC NON-TOUCH TECHNIQUE

The non-touch principle requires not touching the key parts and key sites. Key parts are the parts of equipment that if contaminated by infectious material, increase the risk of infection to the patient. Table 1.4 shows eight key parts.

The 13 principles of ANTT are:

1. **Correct hand hygiene:** infection control principles start with correct hand washing.
2. **Correct use of personal protection equipment** (PPE): PPE includes gowns, gloves, aprons, goggles and visors.
3. **Correct preparation of the environment:** worktops and surfaces should be cleaned using the 'S' technique, which means wiping from side to side so as not to recontaminate areas.
4. **Correct preparation of aseptic field:** clean trolleys and trays may act as your aseptic field.
5. **Correct preparation of equipment:** packaging should be removed and disposed of outside your aseptic field.
6. **Protect key parts (i):** key parts should not be contaminated. Contamination is avoided by using the 'non-touch' technique.

Table 1.4 Key parts of equipment.

Key part	Information
Syringe tip	Should be protected at all times, as it is the key part. If this key site is contaminated, it may result in a healthcare acquired infection (HCAI).
Hub of needles	Should be protected, as it will come into contact with the syringe tip (another key part).
Rubber bungs of drug ampoules	A key part that needs to be cleaned with an approved agent, as it is not sterile. Once cleaned, only the key part of the needle shaft should come into contact with the rubber bung.
Venepuncture needles	A key part that should not be touched or contaminated as it is puncturing the patient's vein.
Intravenous (IV) administration sets – spike	A key part that should not be contaminated as it is penetrating the infusate being administered to the patient. If contaminated, it could also contaminate the infusate, putting the patient at risk of an HCAI.
IV administration sets – connector	A key part, being attached to a needle-free device. It should not be touched or contaminated and should only come into contact with other key parts/sites.
Peripheral venous cannula	A key part that should not be touched or contaminated as it is puncturing the patient's vein.
Dressings	A key part that should not be touched or contaminated before or during applying the dressing to a wound, as contamination can cause an HCAI.

7. **Correct disposal of PPE:** gloves, aprons etc. should be disposed of in the correct waste disposal.
8. **Rewash or gel hands:** prior to the procedure.
9. **Reapply PPE:** gloves, aprons etc.
10. **Prepare patient:** this includes correct identification of the patient, checking allergies and gaining consent.
11. **Protect key parts (ii):** key parts should not be contaminated. Contamination is avoided by using the 'non-touch' technique.
12. **Dispose of PPE:** used PPE should be disposed of in the correct waste disposal.
13. **Clean and store equipment:** all equipment should be stored away after being cleaned.

To help our understanding, have a go at Activity 1.1. Decide whether you would wear sterile or non-sterile gloves and put a tick in the correct column, and whether the skill is an aseptic, aseptic non-touch or clean technique.

ACTIVITY

Activity 1.1

Clinical activity	Sterile gloves	Non-sterile gloves	Aseptic, ANTT or clean technique?
Providing mouth care to the unconscious patient			
Inserting a urinary catheter			
Preparing intravenous medications			
Emptying a urinary catheter			
Emptying a urinal full of urine			
Emptying a commode full of faeces			
Inserting a cannula into a patient's hand			
Taking blood via venepuncture			
Changing a tracheostomy stoma dressing			
Changing a surgical wound site			

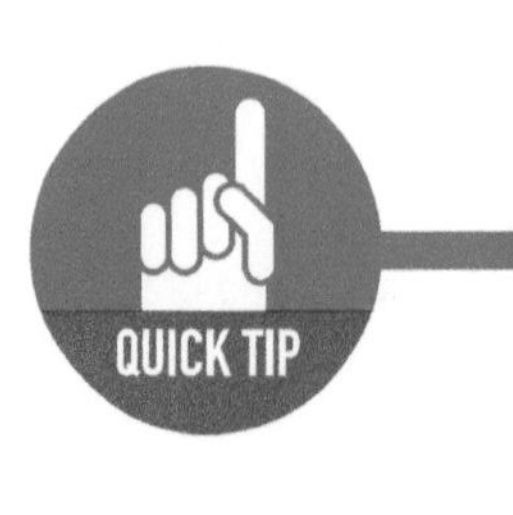

How to remember the ANTT principles using an acronym

A Always wash hands
N Non-touch technique to protect key parts
T Touch non-key parts with confidence
T Take appropriate infection prevention precautions

CORRECT USE OF PPE

Principle 2 of ANTT is the correct use of PPE. PPE covers the use of disposable gowns, aprons, masks, goggles/visors and gloves, and is covered by the Health & Safety at Work Act 1974 etc. PPE should be easily accessible for all staff in their working environment.

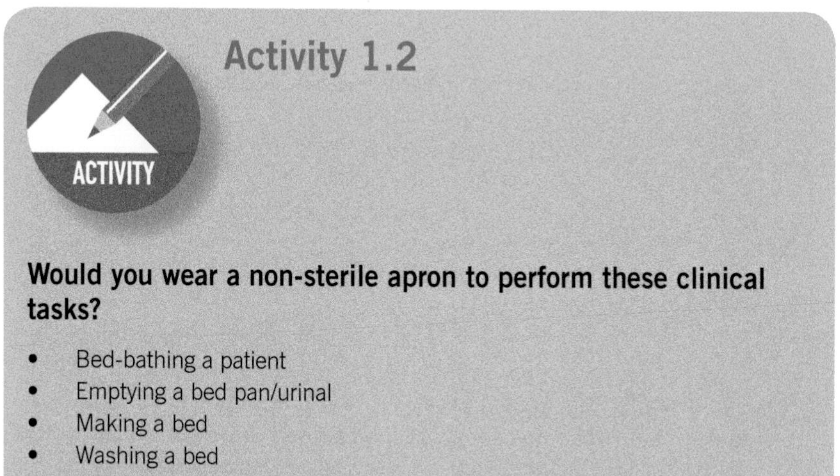

Activity 1.2

Would you wear a non-sterile apron to perform these clinical tasks?

- Bed-bathing a patient
- Emptying a bed pan/urinal
- Making a bed
- Washing a bed
- Changing a stoma bag
- Cleaning a trolley
- Cleaning a drip stand
- Inserting a peripheral cannula

Removing Peripheral Cannulas

Putting into practice what we know about ANTT, the next section shows us how to remove a peripheral cannula using a clean technique avoiding touching key parts while wearing non-sterile gloves and disposable apron.

Equipment:

- Clean surface – dressing trolley or tray
- Disposable plastic apron
- Non-sterile gloves
- Sterile gauze

- Sterile plaster (or other covering if patient is allergic to plaster)
- Yellow sharps bin
- Clinical waste bag
- Alcohol hand rub

Steps:

1. Explain the procedure to the patient and obtain consent.
2. Clean hands correctly with soap and water or alcohol hand rub.
3. Apply non-sterile gloves and apron.
4. Clean tray with chlorhexidine and alcohol wipe.
5. Open sterile gauze packaging and leave gauze in packaging.
6. Take equipment to patient's bedside.
7. Remove gloves/apron and dispose of.
8. Clean hands with soap and water or alcohol hand rub.
9. Apply non-sterile gloves and apron.
10. Loosen existing cannula dressing gently.
11. Remove gauze from packet touching one side only and place over cannula site – do not apply pressure or push down on gauze.
12. Slowly remove the cannula and dressing (checking whole unit integrity) and dispose of in sharps bin.
13. Once cannula is removed, apply pressure to gauze until haemostasis is achieved. Check cannula site.
14. Apply plaster (or other covering) until puncture site is closed.
15. Remove gloves and apron.
16. Clean hands with soap and water or alcohol hand rub.
17. Document that the cannula has been removed.

Now be honest, how many of us have seen healthcare staff taking peripheral cannulas out with no PPE on and not even taking a sharps bin for the safe disposal of sharps. This brings me back to the start of this chapter: as our knowledge in infection control principles have increased, our execution of this knowledge still needs to be addressed.

TEST YOUR KNOWLEDGE

1. What is the definition of asepsis?
2. True or false – an aseptic field can be left unattended for up to two hours?
3. Can you touch key parts and key sites if you are wearing gloves?
4. Can you touch key parts and key sites if you are not wearing gloves?
5. When preparing intravenous medications, what type of technique is used and what type of gloves should be worn?
6. When emptying a commode full of faeces, what type of technique is used and what type of gloves should be worn?
7. What is the second principle of ANTT?
8. True or false – the rubber bung of a drug ampoule is a key part.
9. True or false – standard ANTT is generally used for procedures involving large open sites.
10. The chain of infection has how many links?

KEY POINTS

- Micro-organisms
- Hand hygiene
- The chain of infection
- ANTT

USEFUL WEB RESOURCES

ANTT: www.antt.org

World Health Organization infection control guidelines: www.infectioncontrolresults.com/the-whos-infection-control-guidelines

Health and Safety at Work Act 1974: https://www.hse.gov.uk/legislation/hswa.htm

NHS healthcare associated infections: https://www.england.nhs.uk/patient-safety/healthcare-associated-infections

National Insitute for Health and Care Excellence guidance on healthcare associated infections: https://www.nice.org.uk/guidance/qs113

Royal College of Nursing *Understanding Aseptic Technique*: https://www.rcn.org.uk/professional-development/publications/pub-007928

Government guidance on healthcare associated infections: https://www.gov.uk/government/collections/healthcare-associated-infections-hcai-guidance-data-and-analysis

REFERENCE

World Health Organization (2009). *Your 5 Moments for Hand Hygiene*. Geneva: WHO Available at https://www.who.int/gpsc/5may/Your_5_Moments_For_Hand_Hygiene_Poster.pdf (accessed 13 January 2022).

Chapter 2

PERFORMING OBSERVATIONS

Clinical Skills for Nurses, Second Edition. Claire Boyd.

LEARNING OUTCOMES

By the end of this chapter you will have an understanding of the theory and practice of performing respiration, oxygen saturations, blood pressure, pulse rate, temperature, and consciousness se clinical observations. You will also have the knowledge of plotting the vital sign scores on the NEWS 2 chart and knowing when to escalate.

Observing patients' vital signs is a fundamental healthcare task. Starting at the beginning, every time a set of observations is taken, valid consent must be obtained from the patient.

CONSENT

When a patient lacks the capacity to consent, as with all clinical skills, observations can be made if the procedure is in the patient's best interests. This is part of the Mental Capacity Act 2005, which is an Act of Parliament. Its primary purpose is to provide a legal framework for acting and making decisions on behalf of adults who lack the capacity to make particular decisions for themselves.

The three key factors when testing for valid consent are:

1. Does the patient have enough information to make the decision?
2. Does the patient have enough capacity to make the decision?
3. Has the patient made a free choice?

All three tests must be met for you to have obtained valid consent.

OBSERVATION CHARTS

Observation charts have changed considerably over time and especially since the introduction of the National Early Warning Score observation chart (NEWS 2). This chart enables us to assess our patients' condition and care for them before it becomes critical. It is important that we understand how to use the NEWS 2 chart, as gathering information is only one part of the vital signs assessment.

The NEWS 2 observation chart can be seen in Appendix 1. The chart records six vital signs (or physiological measurements) in the order of A, B, C, D, and E:

A and B	**Relates to the patient's respiration rate (RR)**
A and B	**Also relates to the patient's oxygen saturations (SpO_2)**
C	**Relates to the systolic blood pressure**
C	**Also relates to the pulse rate (also referred to as the heart rate)**
D	**Relates to the patient's consciousness or any new confusion**
E	**Relates to the patient's temperature**

The NEWS 2 observation chart can be used on:

- all adult in-patients (and care home residents)
- occasionally, children in adult wards
- pregnant mothers up to 20 weeks.

There are also adapted NEWS 2 charts for patients requiring neurological observations, which have the Glasgow Coma Scale (GCS) incorporated into the chart, which we look at in Chapter 3. There are also adapted charts for use in maternity (for pregnant mothers over 20 weeks of gestation), children, babies and neonates, and for patients requiring-end-of-life care.

The NEWS 2 chart is brightly coloured; each vital sign generates a score of 0–3, depending on which colour zone the recording is plotted:

White	**Scores 0 (zero)**
Yellow	**Scores 1**
Orange	**Scores 2**
Red	**Scores 3**

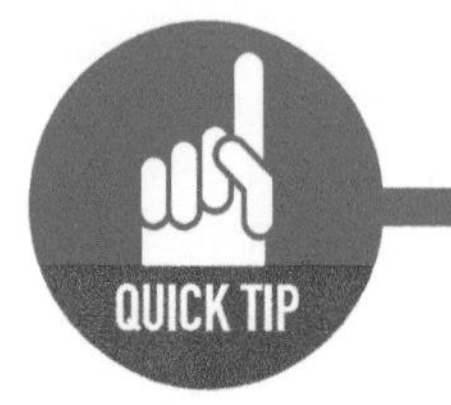

Remember: red means danger and if any recording is placed in the red section, a doctor must be informed at once.

Once all the vital sign scores have been collected and plotted on the chart and totted up to give a score, we are directed as to what to do with this information:

- A total score of 0 directs that we should continue to monitor the patient for a minimum of 12 hours.
- A total score of 1–4 directs that we should continue to monitor the patient for a minimum of four to six hours.
- A score of 3 in any single parameter directs us to continue to monitor the patient once hourly and to inform the nurse in charge and the doctor.
- A score of 5 or more directs us to continue to monitor the patient once hourly and to obtain an urgent medical review.
- A total score of 7 or more directs us to obtain an emergency medical assessment.

For a fuller account on how to use the NEWS 2 chart, the website details have been added at the end of the chapter.

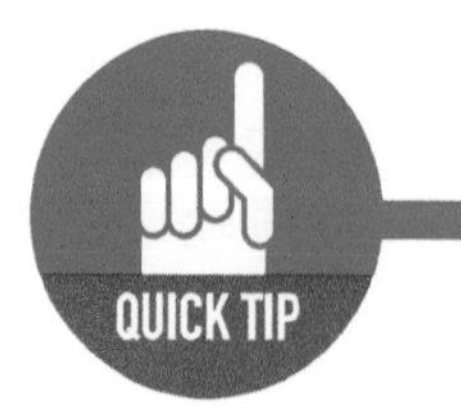

Claire's calculations book in the Student Survival Series explains how to use the NEWS 2 chart more in depth and has loads of examples to work out.

VITAL SIGNS

We start with the basic vital signs, looking at how to gather the recordings to plot on our chart.

All patients admitted to hospital should have a 'manual' set of essential observations recorded; this is known as a **baseline**. Any changes to this norm will trigger action. Of course, the patient could be so ill as to present with a set of abnormal readings, but it is still important to monitor the patient on admission so that we can see when progress is being made with their condition.

BODY TEMPERATURE

Body temperature is measured using a calibrated clinical electronic thermometer or tympanic thermometer. In children's nursing, 'smart-material' tempo dot thermometer strips are often used (Figure 2.1). Mercury glass thermometers are used very rarely in hospitals today. It is considered best practice to document the temperature recording on the observation chart as a solid dot, connecting these dots with a straight line. This is the same procedure as for documented recordings of all vital signs.

Tympanic membrane
The membrane in the eardrum that separates the outer and middle ears.

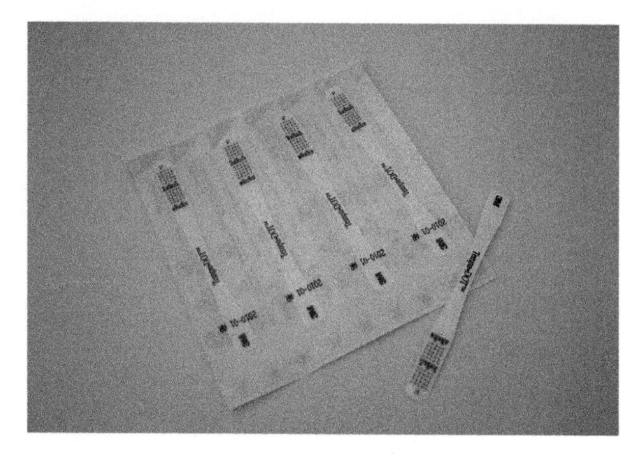

Figure 2.1 Tempo dot thermometer strips.

The sites for recording body temperature are:

- **Oral:** the thermometer is placed in the posterior sublingual pocket, situated at the base of the tongue.
- **Axilla:** the thermometer is placed in the centre of the armpit, with the patient's arm lying across their chest. The same site should be used for all recordings; that is, do not change armpits.
- **Rectum:** a special thermometer is inserted at least 4 cm into the anus of an adult, or 2–3 cm in infants. This provides the most accurate reading of all sites. Rectal temperature readings are usually about 1°C higher than readings taken in the ear.
- **Ear:** to take a temperature reading in the ear, a device known as a tympanic membrane thermometer (Figure 2.2), which is covered with a disposable cuff, is inserted snugly into the ear canal. These devices use infrared light to measure body temperature. The same ear should be used each time for consistent results. Some clinical areas have reconfigured the display screen to show the oral temperature but the device must still be placed in the ear.

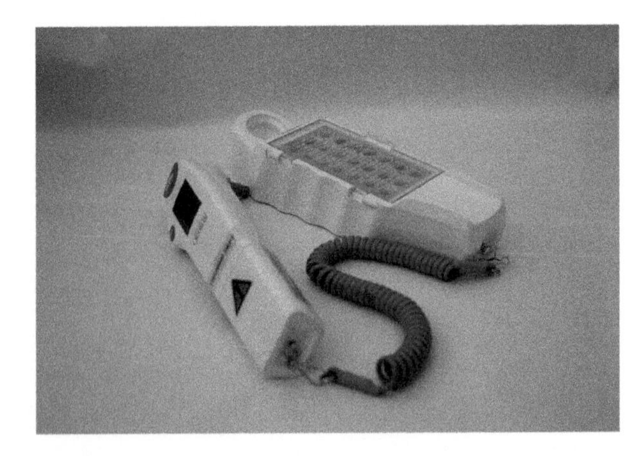

Figure 2.2 A tympanic membrane thermometer.

Single-use plastic-coated 'smart-material' strips are also used, often in paediatric care, which have heat-sensitive dots that change colour to indicate the temperature (Figure 2.1). The strip can be placed across the forehead or in the mouth.

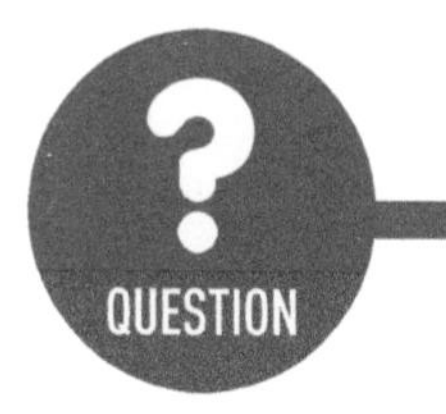

Question 2.1 What are the reasons for recording an individual's body temperature? List five, reasons if you can.

Body Temperature Physiology

Body temperature is usually maintained between 36 and 37.5°C. A body temperature well above the normal range (41°C) is called **hyperthermia** and can result in convulsions. A temperature below normal temperature (35°C) is called **hypothermia** (Table 2.1).

Pyrexia is defined as a rise in body temperature above the normal, usually caused by a viral or bacterial infection. Lay person's terminology for this is 'having a temperature' (Table 2.2).

Table 2.1 Hyperthermia and hypothermia.

Condition	Possible causes
Hyperthermia	Heat stroke, malignancy, stroke, central nervous system damage
Hypothermia	Environmental exposure, medication and exposure of body and internal organs during surgery

Table 2.2 Pyrexia.

Pyrexia grade	Temperature (°C)
Low	Normal – 38
Moderate to high	38–40
Hyperpyrexia	≥ 40

Procedure for Obtaining a Patient's Temperature Using a Tympanic Membrane Thermometer

In many clinical areas, staff *must* have undertaken training in the use of this equipment.

1. Explain and discuss the procedure with the patient. Gain consent.
2. Wash your hands.
3. Check which ear is being used for the reading.
4. Remove thermometer from the base unit and ensure the device is clean (Figure 2.2).
5. Place a disposable probe cover on the probe tip.
6. Gently place the probe tip in the ear canal to seal the opening, ensuring a snug fit.
7. As soon as device indicates (usually by bleeping) that the temperature has registered, remove it from the ear.
8. Press the release/eject button on the device to remove the probe cover.
9. Replace the thermometer in its base unit.
10. Record the reading on the patient's observation chart.

Documenting a Temperature Reading on an Observation Chart

Let's look at the observation chart (Appendix 1). Just for the moment, we will keep it simple. Let's say our patient has a temperature of 36.5°C, this is in the white section of the chart and scores 0. If this same patient had a score of 39.0°C, it would be in the orange-coloured section and would generate a score of 2.

Of course, we would always do a full set of observations and tot up the scores for all the vital signs to get our final NEWS 2 score, not just the temperature recording in isolation.

DID YOU KNOW?

Student nurse: Did you know, it was Daniel Gabriel Fahrenheit and Anders Celsius who named the terms we use for thermometer scales?

Nursing associate: Don't you think it's a bit egocentric to name it after yourself?

Student nurse: Well, to be fair, they both worked hard for their degrees!

BLOOD PRESSURE

Blood pressure is the force extended by the blood as it flows through the blood vessels. Blood pressure increases with age, weight gain, stress and anxiety. Normal range for an adult is usually considered to be 100/60–140/90 mmHg. The first figure is known as the **systolic** reading and the second figure is the **diastolic** reading. Although we record both figures on our observation chart, it is only the systolic reading that generates a score. Table 2.3 lists some of the terms you may hear in relation to the blood pressure reading.

Of course, we should never lose sight of the fact that we are all individuals and have our own 'normal' range for the vital signs.

Blood Pressure Equipment

Increasingly electronic sphygmomanometers (also known as automatic or oscillometric machinery; Figure 2.3) are being used to monitor blood pressure, but these may not achieve the same level of accuracy as manual sphygmomanometers (also known as aneroid sphygmomanometers);

Table 2.3 Terms related to the blood pressure reading.

Normotension	**Blood pressure within normal range**
Hypotension	**Blood pressure lower than normal range**
Hypertension	**Blood pressure higher than normal range**

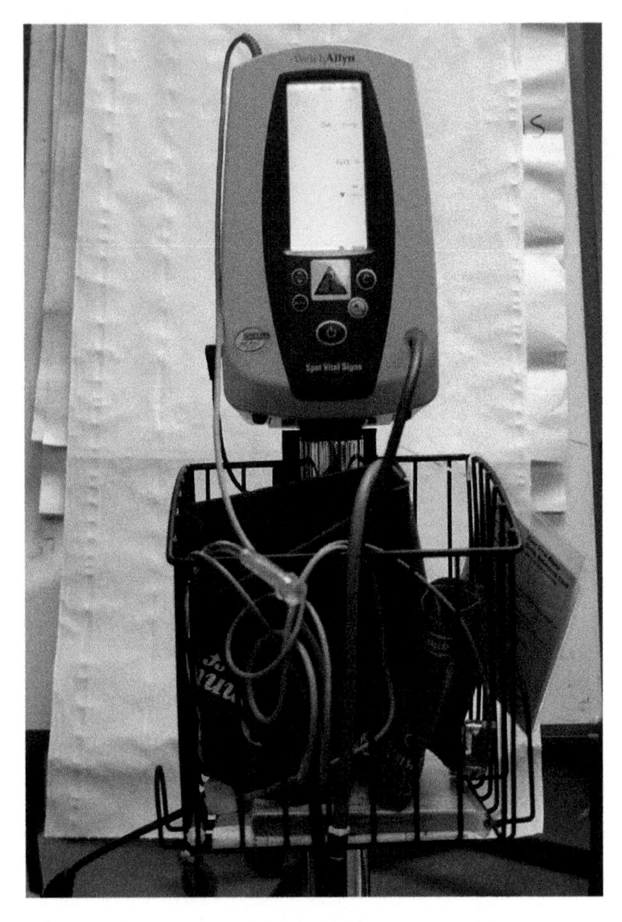

Figure 2.3 An automated blood pressure machine.

Figure 2.4). This is especially so in certain disease states, such as arrhythmias, pre-eclampsia and certain vascular diseases. Staff using these machines should be trained and assessed on how to use them correctly.

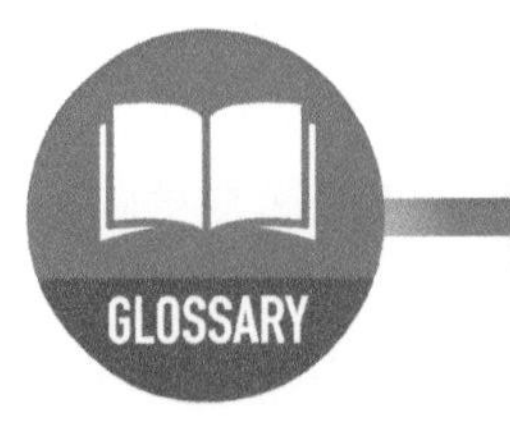

Sphygmomanometer

An instrument for measuring the blood pressure in the arteries.

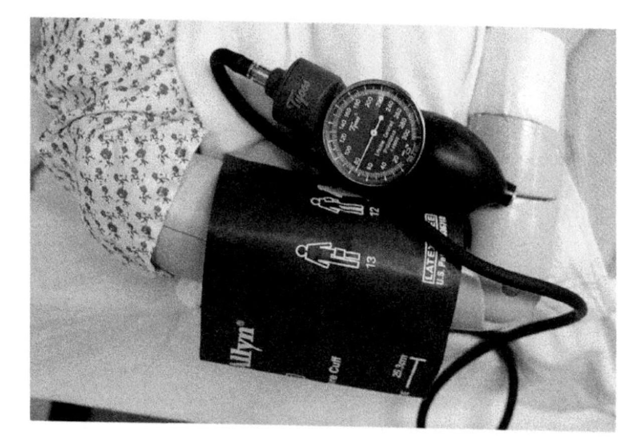

Figure 2.4 An aneroid sphygmomanometer.

Automated blood pressure machines should also not be used on patients with irregular heart rates or on patients with movement disorders, such as Parkinsonian tremors. These patients' blood pressure recordings should be taken using a manual aneroid sphygmomanometer and stethoscope, which you will be shown how to use during your nurse training.

Medics may occasionally request that patients have a 'lying and standing' blood pressure recording, and this is exactly as it sounds: taking the blood pressure first while the patient is lying down, then when standing. Beware that the patient may experience postural hypotension and may feel dizzy when standing.

Which arm was used to record the blood pressure should be documented in the care plan, to avoid variations in reading and consistency. Blood pressures should not be taken from a patient's arms that are affected by arterio-venous fistulae, paralysis or breast surgery, or in which intravenous (IV) lines are situated.

Blood pressure cuffs should be the appropriate size to fit the patient, to ensure accurate measurement. The cuff should cover 80% of the circumference of the upper arm or appropriate limb and should be checked for latex if using on a latex-sensitive individual. Many latex-free cuffs are now available as we are more aware of latex sensitivity. These cuffs should also be wiped clean between patient use to avoid cross-contamination.

Some clinical areas may still have mercury sphygmomanometers, but these are being used much less frequently today because of the dangers of mercury spillage.

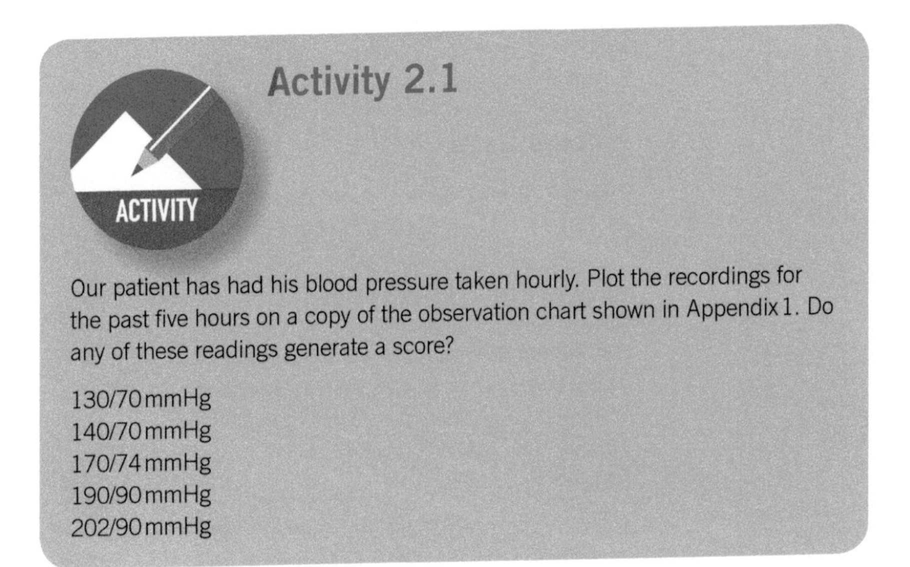

Activity 2.1

Our patient has had his blood pressure taken hourly. Plot the recordings for the past five hours on a copy of the observation chart shown in Appendix 1. Do any of these readings generate a score?

130/70 mmHg
140/70 mmHg
170/74 mmHg
190/90 mmHg
202/90 mmHg

Procedure to Obtain Blood Pressure Using an Aneroid Sphygmomanometer and Stethoscope

You will be shown how to perform this skill during your training, so don't worry if you don't understand the procedure yet. You will need plenty of practice.

1. Wash your hands.
2. Explain procedure to the patient and gain their consent.
3. Gather equipment and clean the stethoscope with an alcohol wipe.

4. Assist the patient into a comfortable position with the arm to be used resting on a firm surface.
5. Roll up the patient's sleeve, making sure that it is not too tight, otherwise this will lead to an inaccurate recording. It may be best to take the arm out of the sleeve if this may be the case.
6. Position the sphygmomanometer at approximately heart level, ensuring that the dial is set at zero.
7. Apply the blood pressure cuff approximately 3–5 cm above where the brachial artery can be palpated (located at the inner side of the biceps). Connect the cuff tubing to the manometer tubing and close the valve to the inflation bulb.
8. Palpate the radial pulse and inflate the cuff until the pulse disappears. Inflate a further 20 mmHg. Release the valve slowly and note when the radial pulse returns. Allow the air to escape from the cuff.
9. Palpate the brachial pulse: Place the stethoscope over the brachial pulse site and inflate the cuff 20 mmHg above the previous reading.
10. Release the valve slowly.
11. When the first pulse is heard, the reading should be noted: *this is the systolic blood pressure.*
12. Continue to deflate the cuff and the pulse will change to a muffled sound until it finally disappears. The reading should be noted: *this is the diastolic blood pressure.*
13. Completely deflate the cuff and remove it from the patient's arm.
14. Clean the stethoscope and cuff.
15. Document the blood pressure recordings and report any abnormalities.
16. Wash your hands.

LYING AND STANDING BLOOD PRESSURE

One of the initiatives to reduce falls in healthcare settings has been the introduction of obtaining a lying and standing blood pressure recording. This is due to the fact that individuals aged 65 years of age and those aged 50–64 years old with underlying medical conditions are more at risk of experiencing a drop in their blood pressure when standing – known as orthostatic hypotension. Before obtaining the lying and standing blood pressure recording, it is important to identify patients who will require assistance to stand. It is also best practice to use a manual sphygmomanometer if possible, and to explain the procedure to the patient first. During the procedure it is important to observe for any symptoms of dizziness, light-headedness, vagueness, pallor, visual disturbances, feelings of weakness, and for any palpitations. These will need to be documented and the medical and nursing teams informed to initiate actions to prevent any falls and/or unsteadiness. The lying and standing blood pressure is conducted as follows:

1. Ask the patient to lie down for at least **five minutes.** Measure the blood pressure.
2. Ask the patient to stand up (assisting if required). Measure the blood pressure after standing up in the **first minute.** Measure it again after the patient has been standing for **three minutes.**
3. Repeat recording if the blood pressure is still dropping. If results are 'positive', repeat regularly until resolved. If symptoms change, repeat the test.

Positive results:

- A drop in systolic blood pressure of 20 mmHg or more (with or without symptoms).
- A drop to below 90 mmHg on standing even if the drop is less than 20 mmHg (with or without symptoms).
- A drop in diastolic blood pressure of 10 mmHg with symptoms (although clinically less significant than a drop in systolic blood pressure).

HEART RATE

Heart rate varies according to age. We can see what the heart rate is by using the pulse rate, which is measured by palpating an artery that lies close to the surface of the body.

Table 2.4 Pulse rates at various ages.

Age	Approximate range (bpm)
Newborn	120–160
1–12 months	80–140
12 months–2 years	80–130
2–6 years	75–120
6–12 years	75–110
Adolescent	60–100
Adult	60–100

The radial artery in the wrist is often the area of choice, due to its accessibility. Normal pulse rates per minute are displayed in Table 2.4.

Heart rate can be felt by feeling the pulse points, so it is sometimes referred to as the pulse rate.

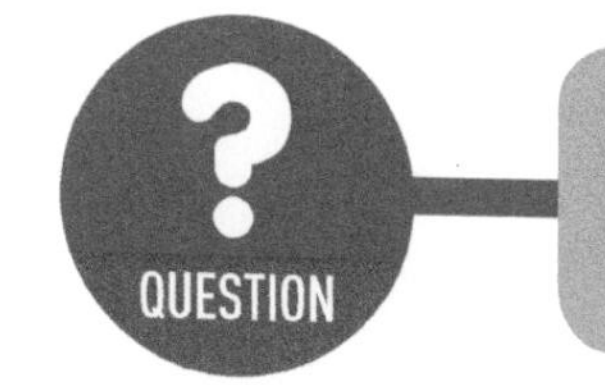

Question 2.2 What are the sites of the major pulse points and where are they located on the body?

The sites of the major pulse points can be viewed in Figure 2.5.

The pulse should be taken for one full minute, assessing for rate, regularity and volume. Patients with a known or suspected irregular heart rate should have a manual reading taken each time this observation is performed.

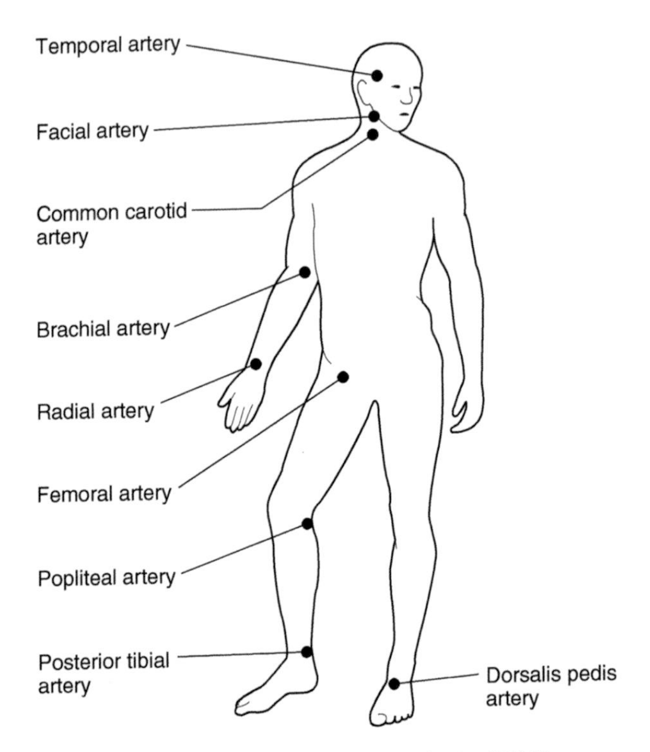

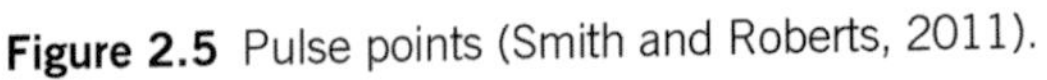
Figure 2.5 Pulse points (Smith and Roberts, 2011).

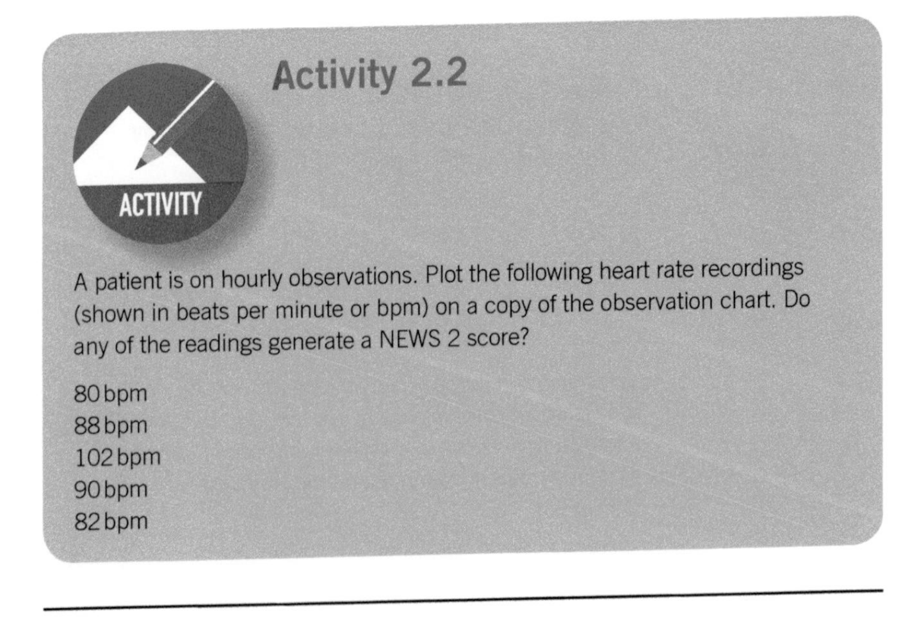

Activity 2.2

A patient is on hourly observations. Plot the following heart rate recordings (shown in beats per minute or bpm) on a copy of the observation chart. Do any of the readings generate a NEWS 2 score?

80 bpm
88 bpm
102 bpm
90 bpm
82 bpm

An abnormally fast heart rate (over 100 bpm in adults) is known as **tachycardia**. This may be caused by raised body temperature, physical/emotional stress or heart disease, as well as certain drugs.

An abnormally slow heart rate (less than 60 bpm) is known as **bradycardia**. This may be caused by low body temperature and certain drugs. Very fit athletes also tend to have low pulse rates.

Procedure to Obtain a Pulse Reading

1. Wash your hands.
2. Explain the procedure to the patient and gain their consent.
3. Locate the radial artery by placing the second and third fingers along it and press gently. Some nurses prefer to use three fingers.
4. Count the pulse for 60 seconds, assessing for rate, regularity and volume.
5. Document the recordings and report any irregularities or abnormalities.
6. Wash your hands.

DID YOU KNOW?

Romeo and Juliet would not have died if Romeo had just taken Juliet's pulse! Doh!

RESPIRATIONS

On the NEWS 2 observation chart, the respiratory rate section is at the top, showing how crucial this recording is. A change in a patient's respiratory rate is a sensitive predictor of deterioration, and can be a precursor to an adverse event, such as a cardiac arrest, up to four hours prior to its occurrence. Trends in respiratory rate on a chart are therefore very important.

The respiratory system supplies the body with oxygen and removes the carbon dioxide through the rhythmic expansion and deflation of the lungs. Each respiration consists of an inhalation, exhalation and pause.

Ventilation is the act of breathing, with air moving in and out of the respiratory tract. Ventilation is under **involuntary control**, being dependent on the respiratory centre in the medulla oblongata and pons varolii, which are situated at the top of the brain stem.

Ventilation is also under **voluntary control** and is regulated through the central nervous system (CNS). The CNS enables individuals to maintain conscious control over their breathing rate.

It is for this reason we should not let patients know when we are counting the rise and fall of their chest (monitoring the **respiratory rate**), as they can alter their natural rhythm as a result.

The respiratory rate is the number of breaths per minute. Normal respiratory rates vary according to age, with the often-accepted normal ranges displayed in Table 2.5.

A good respiratory assessment should be assessed over one full minute, and includes looking, and reporting on:

- the *rate* of breathing: regular or irregular
- the *depth* of breathing: normal, shallow or deep
- the *patient's colour*: pink, flushed, cyanosed
- the *sounds* and *ease* of breathing: effortless, laboured, noisy, abnormal.

Table 2.5 Respiratory rate in various age groups.

Age group	Approximate range (breaths per minute)
Healthy adults	12–20
Adolescents	18–22
Children	22–28
Infants	≥ 30

Table 2.6 Abnormal patterns of breathing.

Pattern	What to look for
Dyspnoea	Difficult, laboured breathing. Shoulders are often raised, nostrils dilated and veins visible in the neck.
Cheyne–Stokes	There is a gradual increase in the depth of respiration followed by a gradual decrease and then a period of no respiration (apnoea). This syndrome is associated with end-of-life care.
Kussmaul's respirations	There is an increased rate and depth of respiration with panting and long grunting expirations. Associated with lobar pneumonia.
Stertorous respirations	Noisy respirations caused by secretions in the trachea or bronchi. May be due to partial airway obstruction.
Stridor	A high-pitched noise heard on inspiration which is caused by laryngeal obstruction. This is a medical emergency.

Abnormal patterns of breathing are described in Table 2.6.

The next activity looks at the terminology you will come across in relation to respirations.

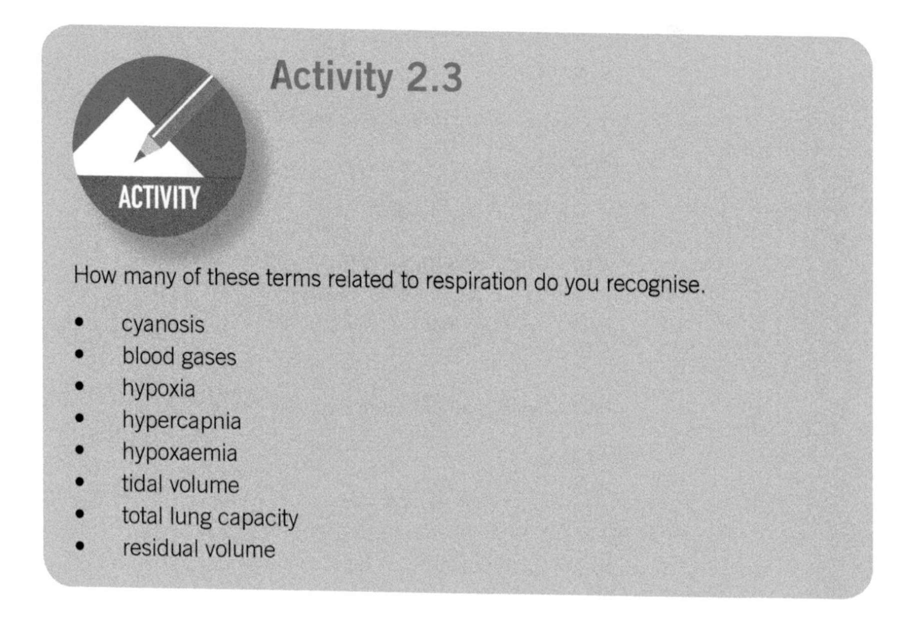

Activity 2.3

How many of these terms related to respiration do you recognise.

- cyanosis
- blood gases
- hypoxia
- hypercapnia
- hypoxaemia
- tidal volume
- total lung capacity
- residual volume

Procedure to Obtain a Reading for Respiratory Rate

1. Ensure that the patient is relaxed and not aware that you are assessing their respirations.
2. Count the respiratory rate and assess the rate, depth and ease of breathing and patient's colour (for cyanosis) for one full minute.
3. Document the recordings and report any abnormal findings.

NEUROLOGICAL OBSERVATIONS

A full neurological assessment is conducted using the GCS. The GCS looks at the patient's level of consciousness, pupillary activity, motor function, sensory function and their vital signs, with each test equating to a score. We look at the GCS in more depth in Chapter 3, where you will be shown how to use the tool.

If you look at the NEWS 2 chart and the consciousness section, you will see ACVPU, which means:

A = alert

C = new confusion

V = patient only responding to verbal stimuli

P = patient only responding to painful stimuli

U = patient unresponsive

Only the 'alert' recording does not generate a trigger or score. If the patient is recorded as C, V, P, or U, we would need to measure their GCS and inform the nurse in charge.

Procedure for Obtaining an ACVPU Recording

Simply approaching our patient and talking to them will tell us if they are alert (A) or responding to voice (V). C is only recorded if the patient shows 'new confusion', as confusion may be their 'norm' (i.e. patients with dementia). If we are required to give them a painful stimulus, this is usually conducted by performing a 'trapezium squeeze'.

The Trapezium Squeeze

Using the thumb and two fingers, hold 5 cm of the trapezium muscle, where the neck and shoulder meet, and twist.

OXYGEN SATURATION

Oxygen saturation (peripheral capillary oxygen saturation or SpO_2) is routinely measured with a pulse oximetry machine, after training and assessment to use this machinery.

Red blood cells contain haemoglobin molecules, which bind with oxygen to form oxyhaemoglobin. Pulse oximetry works on the principle that blood saturated with oxygen is a different colour from deoxygenated blood. The clean probe, which is placed on a finger, contains a light source and detector, which shines through the tissues of the body to obtain the oxygen saturation reading.

The pulse oximeter will not display a correct estimate of the oxygen saturation unless the machine is able to accurately capture the patient's pulse reading. The user should always check the patient's manual pulse against the waveform displayed by the machine.

Pulse oximeters will not give accurate measurements if the patient is peripherally compromised, is wearing nail varnish, or has a dark skin, as this interferes with the light source on the probe. Bright or fluorescent room lighting may also interfere with the light transmission on the probe. Pulse detection on the probe may be interfered with by patient movement (such as Parkinsonian movement disorders), rigors or shivering.

Owing to the limitations with this machinery, the pulse oximeter should not replace either the manual respiratory rate or pulse measurement.

Part of the A and B section of the NEWS 2 chart assesses the oxygen saturation using two different target scales:

- Scale 1 is used for patients who are not at risk of hypercapnic failure.
- Scale 2 is used for patients with or *at high risk of* hypercapnic failure.

Only a doctor, nurse practitioner or specialised nurse from the respiratory team can generally authorise the use of scale 2. An extra score of 2 is added for patients requiring supplementary oxygen. The codes for the oxygen administration device should also be recorded on the NEWS 2 chart, as seen in Table 2.7.

Table 2.7 Oxygen device codes.

Code	Device
A	**Air**
NC	**Nasal cannula**
SM	**Simple mask**
RM	**Reservoir mask**
VM	**Venturi mask**
TM	**Tracheostomy mask**
CH	**Cold humidified**
HH	**Heated humidified**
CP	**CPap (continuous positive airway pressure)**
BP	**BiPap (bi-level positive airway pressure)**
HFNO	**High-flow nasal oxygen**

TEST YOUR KNOWLEDGE

1. Go back to the NEWS 2 observation chart in Appendix 1 and input these observations from a patient. What is this patient's NEWS? What would be your actions?
   - Respiratory rate: 30 breaths per minute
   - Oxygen saturation, SpO_2 95% scale 1, supplementary oxygen
   - Blood pressure: 192/74 mmHg
   - Heart rate: 110 bpm
   - Neurological response: alert
   - Temperature: 38.4°C
2. What does the code TM mean in relation to the oxygen administration device?
3. If a patient scores 3 in any of the coloured zones on the NEWS 2 chart, what are your actions?
4. What is the approximate pulse range of a newborn baby?
5. What is the name for a drop in the blood pressure on standing?
6. What does 'C' stand for in relation to the ACVPU neurological assessment?

KEY POINTS

- Obtaining valid consent.
- Using the NEWS 2 observation chart.
- Performing vital sign observations of temperature, blood pressure, heart rate, respiration, neurological indicators and oxygen saturation.

USEFUL WEB RESOURCES

Royal College of Physicians. National Early Warning Score (NEWS) 2: https://www.rcplondon.ac.uk/projects/outputs/national-early-warning-score-news

Royal College of Physicians. Measurement of lying and standing blood pressure: a brief guide for clinical staff: https://www.rcplondon.ac.uk/projects/outputs/measurement-lying-and-standing-blood-pressure-brief-guide-clinical-staff

Royal Children's Hospital Melbourne. Observation and continuous monitoring: https://www.rch.org.au/rchcpg/hospital_clinical_guideline_index/Observation_and_continuous_monitoring

REFERENCE

Smith, J. and Roberts, R. (2011). *Vital Signs for Nurses: An introduction to clinical observations*. Chichester: Wiley.

Chapter 3

ABCDE ASSESSMENT

LEARNING OUTCOMES

By the end of this chapter you will have an understanding of the theory and practice of performing the clinical skill of conducting an ABCDE assessment and escalating our concerns.

Chapter 1 showed us how to perform vital signs observations. Now we need to know what to do with the information we have obtained, and how best to communicate our concerns to the nurse in charge and/or to medics in more detail. This is undertaken using the situation, background, assessment, recommendation (SBAR) communication tool.

SITUATION, BACKGROUND, ASSESSMENT, RECOMMENDATION

Situation, background, assessment, recommendation (SBAR) is a communication tool referred to as 'critical language'. The tool is used in the airline industry, whereby key phrases are understood by all to mean 'stop and listen to me – we have a potential problem'. Put simply, this is:

> 'Doctor, I'm concerned about Patient A and would like you to review her immediately.'

Of course, medics require more information than this and this is where we get the 'SBAR' bit from:

- S: punchline to be given in 5–10 seconds. No waffling.
- B: how did we get here? Admitting diagnosis. Medical history.
- A: what is the problem? Give ABCDE recording results.
- R: what do we need to do?

Here is an example of how the tool is used in practice, and the score it generates in conjunction with the National Early Warning Score (NEWS2) chart in Appendix 1:

Identify yourself and clinical area first. 'Doctor, I'm concerned about Patient A, who was admitted this morning with a chest infection. I have just assessed her and her vital signs are: respirations 30 breaths per minute (3), oxygen saturation (SpO_2) on scale one is 90% on 2 l of oxygen therapy (nasal cannula) (3 + 2), blood pressure 192/74 (0), pulse 110 bpm irregular (2), ACVPU is V (3). Temperature 38.4°C (2); her NEWS 2 Score is 15. I have increased her oxygen therapy (non-rebreather mask) and arranged for an ECG recording. I will site a peripheral venous access device. I would like you to review her immediately.'

Using the SBAR communication tool really does stop you from panicking and keeps you focused. During this communication all the bases were covered: the SBAR. Each of the red numbers is the score generated from the patient's vital signs. Let's look at this in more detail.

NATIONAL EARLY WARNING SCORE

We looked at the NEWS 2 observation Chart in Chapter 2 (see also Appendix 1). We know that each vital sign on the chart generates a score from 0 to 3. A score of 2 and above generates a *trigger* for action to be implemented, and the second page of the chart shows what action needs to be taken. A score of 4 and above tells us that our patient is quite sick and requires an urgent review by the medics.

When speaking to a medic we would use the SBAR communication tool, using concise and relevant language to convey our concerns. Now you can see how the NEWS 2 chart and SBAR are important tools in improving our response to vital signs when a patient first starts to deteriorate.

On page two of the chart, which you can view by accessing the website at the end of this chapter, is a box saying, 'revised trigger'. This is where a consultant or registrar can adjust the trigger score, initiating a response by the care team. This means that where there is usually a call for action on a score of 2 and above, we may now only be required to do this on a score of 4.

Activity 3.1

ACTIVITY

Here's some practice at using the NEWS 2 observation chart. You are looking after Sandra Singh. She is 65 years of age and had a section of her bowel removed three days ago due to a cancerous tumour. She has been stable postoperatively and has not encountered any major problems. She now has a temporary colostomy, which is functioning. She has non-insulin-dependent diabetes. Her NEWS 2 score has been 0 and her blood glucose levels have been stable.

Sandra is now due her four-hourly observations. Plot them on a copy of the chart. Her blood glucose is 6.2 mmol/l. What is her NEWS 2 score? What are your actions, if any?

- Respiratory rate: 23 breaths per minute
- Oxygen saturation, SpO_2: 92% (on air) scale 1
- Blood pressure: 88/50 mmHg
- Heart rate: 115 bpm (tachycardia)
- Neurological response: verbal
- Temperature: 37.8°C

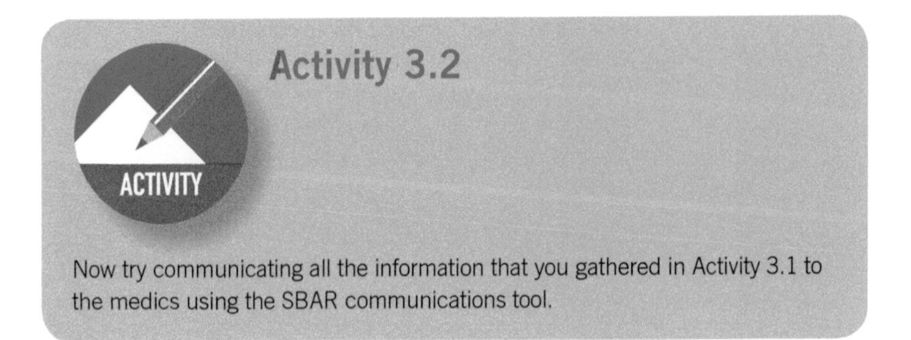

Activity 3.2

ACTIVITY

Now try communicating all the information that you gathered in Activity 3.1 to the medics using the SBAR communications tool.

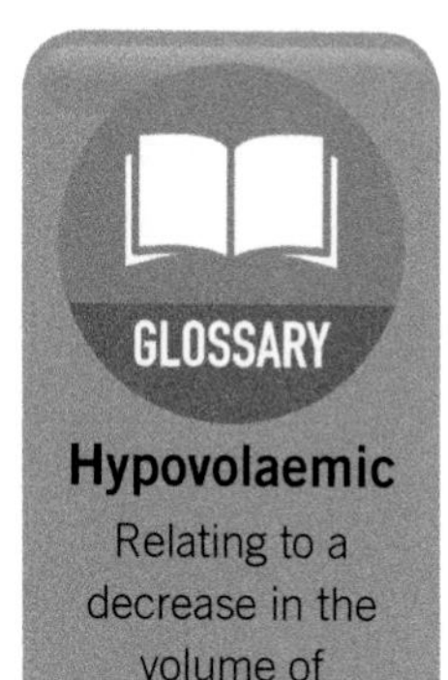

Hypovolaemic

Relating to a decrease in the volume of circulating blood.

EARLY PATIENT ASSESSMENT AND RESPONSE

Did you wonder why Sandra Singh, in Activity 3.1, had started to deteriorate so quickly? She had been sitting up and chatting just one hour previously (and boy, can she chat!) and now was only responsive to verbal neurological observations. Well, this was because no one had looked at her wound site (the colostomy) and noticed that she was bleeding profusely from it, and that she was actually hypovolaemic, hence the drop in blood pressure and increase in heart rate.

If you have undertaken basic first aid you may have used the ABC approach, but in health care today we undertake the ABCDE assessment:

A airway
B breathing
C circulation (including cannulation)
D disability and diuresis (drugs and diabetes)
E expose and early call for help using SBAR

Airway

The first assessment we perform on our patient is the airway. If the airway is occluded, our patient will die, so we will need to address this immediately and clear the obstruction. We need to check that our patient can talk either normally, in sentences, in words, or whether they are unable to talk or are unresponsive. The assessment includes:

- *looking:* any obvious obstruction such as vomit or foreign objects?
- *feeling:* is the chest rising and falling?
- *listening:* can the patient speak? Any gurgling, wheezing or stridor?
- *smelling:* any smell of alcohol, solvents or ketones?

If the patient is expectorating sputum, this is part of the airway assessment. We need to report on the colour, odour, consistency and amount.

When we are satisfied that the airway is clear we can move on to the breathing assessment.

Breathing

Breathing assessment consists of measuring the respiratory rate. Signs of respiratory deterioration include:

- increased respiratory rate (especially if above 30 breaths per minute)
- oxygen decrease by 3%
- increasing oxygen requirements
- increasing NEWS score
- carbon dioxide retention with blood pH below 7.35
- drowsiness
- headache
- tremor.

The breathing assessment requires us to look at the patient for signs of cyanosis around the lips, oral mucosa and nails. We need to observe the depth of breathing and to look for any 'see-saw' chest movements (which may be a sign of a pneumothorax) and for oedema around the face, which may be interfering with the airway.

Our patient may be experiencing dyspnoea with shortness of breath and will assume a position that best facilitates lung expansion: sat forward in their chair, arching back, breathing through the mouth, shoulders forward and nostrils flaring.

If the breathing assessment has not triggered any action based on the NEWS score, or any concerns, we can move on to circulation.

Circulation

Assessment of circulation includes monitoring the pulse (heart rate) and blood pressure. If our patient is experiencing chest pain, and after we have contacted the medics, we may need to conduct an electrocardiogram (ECG). The ECG can tell us (in ST elevation) whether muscle damage has occurred, or if ischaemia has occurred (in ST depression). We look at ECGs in Chapter 16.

The doctor may wish the patient to have intravenous (IV) access, so a cannula may need to be inserted for crystalloid/

colloid fluids to be administered, and other IV drugs. We look at IVs in Chapter 13.

A **capillary refill** test may be conducted. This test measures the rate at which blood refills empty capillaries. To carry out this test:

1. Press firmly on a fingernail to blanch it and count the time it takes for blood to return after the pressure is released.
2. In a normal person, with good cardiac output and digital profusion, capillary refill should take less than two seconds.
3. A time of more than two seconds is considered a sign of sluggish digital circulation.
4. A time of five seconds is considered abnormal.

If the circulation assessment has not triggered any action based on the NEWS score, or any concerns, we can move on to disability.

Disability

Disability assessment has four parts and concerns making neurological observations (the disability component), as well as diuresis, drugs and diabetes.

On our NEWS 2 chart, if our patient has recorded anything other than alert in the neurological response section we need to conduct a full Glasgow Coma Scale (GCS) assessment.

There are many causes of altered consciousness; Table 3.1 shows some of them.

Figure 3.1 shows an example of a neurological observation chart, incorporating the GCS and NEWS 2 systems. In short, the GCS looks at the responses of:

- eye opening
- motor response
- verbal response.

The neurological observation chart also has *limb movement* and *pupillary assessment* sections. At the bottom of the

Table 3.1 Causes of altered consciousness.

Profound hypoxaemia	Cerebral hypoperfusion
Hypercapnia	Stroke
Convulsions	Sedatives
Head injury	Hypoglycaemia
Alcohol intoxication	Analgesic drugs
Subarachnoid haemorrhage	Drug overdose

chart, there are instructions on what to do if the neurological examination is abnormal, the NEWS score to add and the actions to take.

Motor Response

The motor response assessment is designed to determine the patient's ability to obey commands and to localise, and to withdraw (or assume abnormal body positions) in response to painful stimuli, such as the trapezium squeeze.

- Score 6 if the patient can obey a command.
- Score 5 if the patient localises to central pain. This means that the patient does not respond to verbal stimuli but purposely moves an arm to remove the cause of a central painful stimulus.
- Score 4 if the patient withdraws from pain. This means that the patient flexes or bends the arm towards the source of pain but fails to locate the source of pain (no wrist rotation).
- Score 3 if the patient flexes to pain. This means that the patient flexes or bends the arm: this is characterised by internal rotation. Appears slower than normal flexion.
- Score 2 if the patient shows extension to pain. This means that the patient extends the arm by straightening the elbow and possibly wrist rotation.
- Score 1 if there is no response to painful stimuli.

Pupillary Assessment

Pupillary assessment is conducted by observing the preassessment size and shape of the pupils and documenting it (in millimetres). The procedure is then conducted as follows:

Neurological Observation Chart GCS

To be used in conjunction with Bristol Observation Chart

Not to be used on Neuroscience wards

Name: ....

Date of Birth: ....

Hospital No.: ....

Ward: ....

Ensure sections shaded grey are completed after discussion with medical staff requesting neurological observations

Reason for undertaking GCS (circle)

Fall with head injury / suspected head injury

Encephalopathy

CNS infection

Date started:

Head injury

Seizure

Other (specify)

Frequency of neuro obs (circle):	half hour	every hour	every 2 hours	every 4 hours (see NICE for head injury)
Neuro obs to continue for (circle):	next 12 hours	24 hours	48 hours	72 hours
Revise EWS (circle):	Yes	No	If Yes trigger new threshold+	

Please enter date and time in boxes below

		Date																									
		Time																									
Glasgow Coma Scale	Eye opening	Spontaneous	4	4	4	4	4	4	4	4	4	4	4	4	4	4	4	4	4	4	4	4	4	4	4	4	4
		To speech	3	3	3	3	3	3	3	3	3	3	3	3	3	3	3	3	3	3	3	3	3	3	3	3	3
		To pain	2	2	2	2	2	2	2	2	2	2	2	2	2	2	2	2	2	2	2	2	2	2	2	2	2
		None	1	1	1	1	1	1	1	1	1	1	1	1	1	1	1	1	1	1	1	1	1	1	1	1	1
	Motor response	Obeys commands	6	6	6	6	6	6	6	6	6	6	6	6	6	6	6	6	6	6	6	6	6	6	6	6	6
		Localises to pain	5	5	5	5	5	5	5	5	5	5	5	5	5	5	5	5	5	5	5	5	5	5	5	5	5
		Flexion	4	4	4	4	4	4	4	4	4	4	4	4	4	4	4	4	4	4	4	4	4	4	4	4	4
		Abnormal flexion	3	3	3	3	3	3	3	3	3	3	3	3	3	3	3	3	3	3	3	3	3	3	3	3	3
		Extension	2	2	2	2	2	2	2	2	2	2	2	2	2	2	2	2	2	2	2	2	2	2	2	2	2
		None	1	1	1	1	1	1	1	1	1	1	1	1	1	1	1	1	1	1	1	1	1	1	1	1	1
	Verbal response	Orientated	5	5	5	5	5	5	5	5	5	5	5	5	5	5	5	5	5	5	5	5	5	5	5	5	5
		Confused	4	4	4	4	4	4	4	4	4	4	4	4	4	4	4	4	4	4	4	4	4	4	4	4	4
		Inappropriate	3	3	3	3	3	3	3	3	3	3	3	3	3	3	3	3	3	3	3	3	3	3	3	3	3
		Sounds	2	2	2	2	2	2	2	2	2	2	2	2	2	2	2	2	2	2	2	2	2	2	2	2	2
		None	1	1	1	1	1	1	1	1	1	1	1	1	1	1	1	1	1	1	1	1	1	1	1	1	1
		Totals																									
Limb movement	Arms	Normal power																									
		Mild weakness																									
		Severe weakness																									
		Spastic flexion																									
		Extension																									
		No response																									
	Legs	Normal power																									
		Mild weakness																									
		Severe weakness																									
		Spastic flexion																									
		Extension																									
		No response																									
		Pupils																									
Pupils scale (mm)		Right pupil size																									
		Right pupil																									
		Left pupil size																									
		Left pupil reaction																									
		Unequal																									
		Total EWS (BOC + Neuro chart)																									

Please circle appropriate score

Any decrease in motor response add 4 to EWS

Place a cross in the box according to limb movement. Record right (R) and left (L) where the two sides are not the same.

\+ Reacts
\- No reaction
C Eyes closed
SL Sluggish

Total EWS Score

Signature

Pupil scale (mm): 8, 7, 6, 5, 4, 3, 2, 1

ACTIONS if Neurological examination abnormal

If decrease in Motor score - add 4 to EWS score and call 6999 for urgent review.

If total GCS drops by 2 points or more - add 4 points to EWS score and call 6999 for urgent review

If total GCS drops by 1 point or more - add 2 points to EWS score. Patient must be reviewed by Nurse in charge and have a medical review.

Any unilateral pupil changes - add 4 to EWS score and call 6999 for urgent review.

Any new limb weakness - add 2 points to EWS score and patient must be reviewed by Nurse in charge and have medical review.

* If head injury suspected, patient requires neurological observations: half hourly for first two hours, hourly for next 4 hours and then 2 hourly if no change.

Figure 3.1 A neurological observation chart. Source: Permission to reproduce this image is granted by North Bristol NHS Trust and University Hospitals Bristol NHS Foundation Trust.

1. Wash your hands.
2. Explain the procedure to the patient (even if they are unconscious).
3. Dim the overhead lighting, if possible.
4. Move a torchlight from the side of the patient's head towards the pupil and note any change in pupil size and speed of reaction (brisk or sluggish).
5. Check for consensual reflex (opposite pupil reaction).
6. Repeat the procedure in the opposite eye.
7. Document.

The patient may require a painful stimulus, when we would record that the patient is opening their eyes to pain, thus scoring 2 on the chart.

The Other Ds

After we have conducted the neurological assessments we also need to look at the other components of the D assessment; that is, *diabetes, drugs* and *diuresis*.

First, we simply conduct a blood glucose test, as the blood glucose level may be a factor in why our patient is deteriorating, even if they are not known to have diabetes. We also look at the drug chart to see if there are any items with a bearing on our patient's condition and seek to establish whether any drugs have been taken.

Now we come to the *diuresis* component. This assessment can be conducted by looking at the patient's fluid chart to check urine output, but this can only be done if they are actually having their fluids documented.

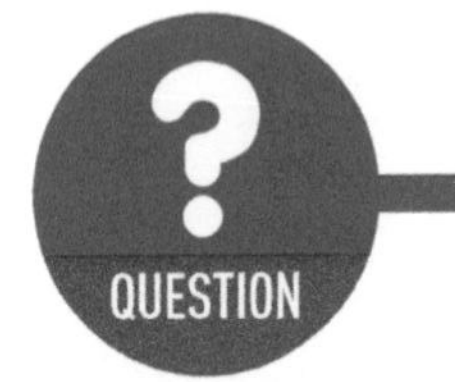

Question 3.1 What do the terms oliguria, anuria and absolute anuria mean?

We would look at our patient's condition as a whole to establish whether the kidneys were being fully perfused, as we know that conditions such as hypovolaemia, hypotension and dehydration would cause ineffective perfusion of the kidneys and have a direct bearing on the urine output. Renal perfusion requires 25% of cardiac output; if our patient had experienced a recent cardiac assault, the renal system would be directly affected. We could also look at our patient's prescription chart, as we know that certain drugs are nephrotoxic; that is, they are associated with structural damage to the nephrons in the kidneys. Some of these drugs include:

- cardiac drugs: angiotensin-converting enzyme inhibitors, beta blockers, radiocontrast media
- non-steroidal anti-inflammatory drugs: diclofenac, ibuprofen
- antibiotics: acyclovir, vancomycin, rifampicin, sulphonamides, ciprofloxacin
- diuretics: furosemide.

If the disability assessment (neurological, blood glucose, diuresis and drugs) has not triggered action based on the NEWS score and there are no other concerns, we can move on to the exposure part of the assessment chain.

Exposure

The exposure assessment is where we literally expose our patient to observe wound sites, etc. The exposure assessment consists of looking for:

- blood or fluid loss
- injuries or foreign objects
- scars (surgical or other)
- skin colour (capillary refill)
- peripheral skin temperature
- distal pulses (femoral/pedal)
- oedema.

We also check the patient's temperature and look at their observations and notes.

Remember Sandra Singh in Activity 3.1? Only when we pulled back her bed clothes did we notice that she was bleeding profusely from her wound site and had actually gone into hypovolaemic shock.

This is how we conduct our ABCDE assessment, which is used in conjunction with NEWS 2 and SBAR to recognise any deterioration in our patients. It allows us to act quickly and efficiently in providing care to reverse the situation, if possible.

CABCDE

In critical care (trauma teams) and the military, the C>ABCDE approach is used:

C Catastrophic haemorrhage
A Airway (with cervical spine control)
B Breathing
C Circulation (with haemorrhage control)
D Disability
E Exposure

The CABCDE framework is about identifying any obvious major bleeding points, such as stab wounds, and immediately applying pressure to stem the flow of blood. This is because bleeding may be the immediate life-threatening issue to deal with so as to preserve life.

In the scenario of Sandra Singh, it would have been the acceptable assessment framework. However, as this patient was on a postoperative ward, the ABCDE framework would have been the most likely one used by the nurses. Remember that not all bleeding is visible, so the vital signs (respirations, heart rate, blood pressure, capillary refill time, mental status and urine output) would have been assessed, as well as the indicators of oxygen deficit (oxygen saturations and venepuncture for lactate, etc). These would have been indicators of the bleed, before we got to the 'exposure' part of the assessment.

TEST YOUR KNOWLEDGE

1 What does SBAR mean?
2 Work out the NEWS 2 score for this patient:
A = 10 breaths per minute, B = oxygen saturations on

scale 1 = 93%, C = blood pressure 210/80 mmHg, C = pulse 90 bpm, D = alert, E = 37.2°C.

3. What are the components of the ABCDE assessment?
4. What is a capillary refill test?

KEY POINTS

- The SBAR communication tool.
- The NEWS 2 system.
- Early patient assessment and response.

USEFUL WEB RESOURCES

Boulanger C, Toghill M. (2009) Practice review: How to measure and record vital signs to ensure detection of deteriorated patients. *Nursing Times* 105: 47: https://www.nursingtimes.net/clinical-archive/critical-care/how-to-meaure-and-record-vital-signs-to-ensure-detection=of-deteriorating-patients

National Institute for Health and Care Excellence. Improving the detection and response to patient deterioration (2011): https://www.nice.org.uk/sharedlearning/improving-the-detection-and-response-to-patient-deterioration

National Institute for Health and Care Excellence. *Acutely Ill Adults in Hospital: Recognising and Responding to Deterioration*. Clinical Guideline CG50 (2007): https://www.nice.org.uk/guidance/CG50

Association of First Air Services. Primary survey trauma: https://aofas.org.uk/primary-survey-trauma

Chapter 4

CONTINENCE CARE

LEARNING OUTCOMES

By the end of this chapter, you will have an understanding of the theory and practice of performing the clinical skill of continence care and knowledge of moisture lesions.

One thing we can all be sure of is that at some point(s) during the day we will all need to void bodily waste by the acts of urination (micturition) or elimination of faeces (or stools); or, to put it in its simplest form, to 'wee and poo'.

URINE

Urine is secreted into the bladder throughout the day but production slows down during sleep. The first void after waking is therefore usually more concentrated and darker in colour. Urine should be what is described as a 'straw-coloured' but it does vary in colour, sometimes being closer to amber.

Urine can also take on other colours due to factors such as disease, medications, fluid intake, infection, trauma or diet.

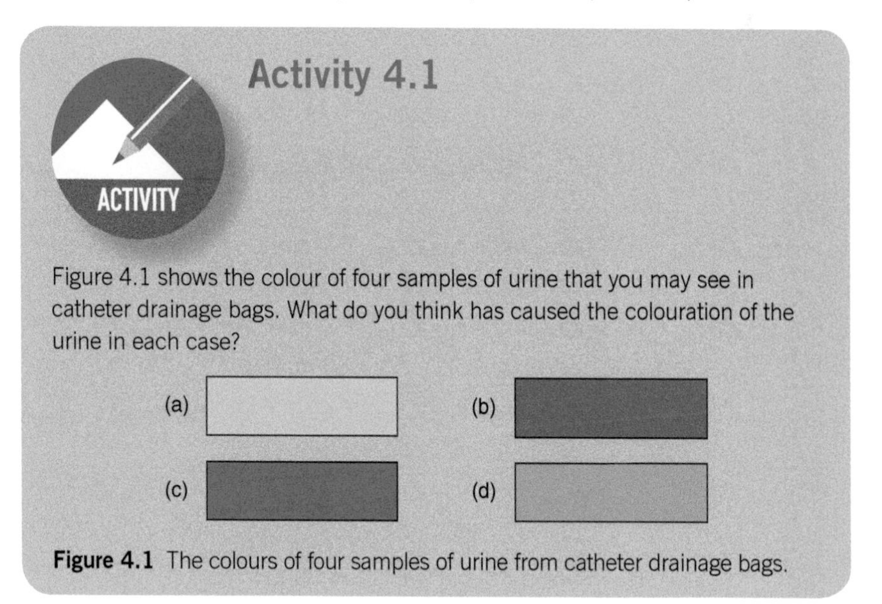

Activity 4.1

Figure 4.1 shows the colour of four samples of urine that you may see in catheter drainage bags. What do you think has caused the colouration of the urine in each case?

Figure 4.1 The colours of four samples of urine from catheter drainage bags.

Question 4.1 What is urine comprised of? Should protein be present in urine?

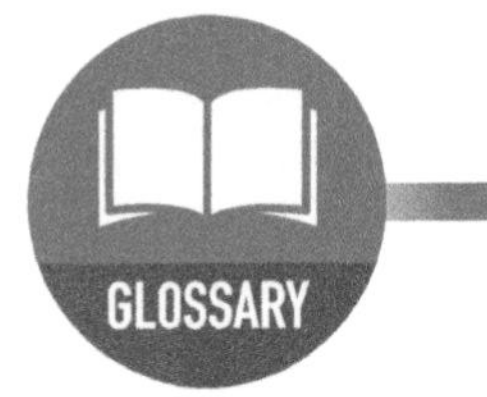

Urinalysis

Also known as a 'urine dipstick' test. A test to establish the pH of urine and what substances or cell types are present, such as protein, glucose, ketones, blood, leucocytes and nitrites.

Urine is mainly made up of water (95%), together with the constituents in Table 4.1. Protein should not be present in urine.

The specific gravity (the relative **density)** of urine is between 1.015 and 1.025. It is acidic in nature, with a pH of about 6 (anything from 4.5 to 8). Drinking more results in a more diluted urine and higher urine output and drinking less leads to a more concentrated urine and decreased urine output.

Table 4.1 Consituents (other than water) of urine.

Constituent	Total in urine (%)
Uric acid	2.0
Potassium	0.6
Chloride	0.6
Sodium	0.1
Creatinine	0.1
Sulphate	0.18
Phosphate	0.12
Ammonia	0.05
Calcium	0.015
Magnesium	0.01

Fresh urine should only have a very slight smell but when it is exposed to air it starts to decomposes and begins to smell very strongly of ammonia.

Micturition or the discharge of urine usually occurs around 5–10 times a day in the average person, who produces about 1–1.5 litres each day. However, I have yet to meet this 'average' person!

When we feel the desire to void, most of us can suppress it for a considerable period of time, until there is a suitable time and place.

Urinary Incontinence

Incontinence is the *involuntary* passing of urine in *inappropriate* places at *inappropriate* times.

Many individuals do not seek help with their urinary incontinence as they often feel too embarrassed about their condition. However, with understanding and careful management, many patients can achieve continence or partial continence. Urinary incontinence is known as **enuresis**.

DID YOU KNOW?

- One person in six over the age of 40 years is incontinent 'several times a month'.
- Incontinence is very common in women after childbirth and during the menopause.
- It is very common in men in later life (especially in those with prostate conditions).

Babies and Children

Newborn babies excrete urine from the urinary bladder after birth as a reflex when the bladder is full. It is an involuntary response. Voluntary control is usually achieved by the age of three years. If healthy children continue to wet themselves after the age of five, or regress to this behaviour pattern after a period of dryness, they are described as experiencing urinary incontinence.

Night-time bed wetting is known as nocturnal enuresis. It is usually treated with a variety of techniques, one of which is based on the conditioning principle. Here, the child is woken during the night and taken to the toilet.

Types and Causes of Urinary Incontinence

When caring for people with urinary incontinence, it is very important that we know what type of urinary incontinence the individual is experiencing so that we can provide the correct care. The term **neurogenic bladder** is used when there is interference with the nerve supply to the bladder, which can result in various forms of incontinence. Six types of urinary incontinence are listed in Table 4.2.

Urinary incontinence can also be a combination of stress and urge incontinence, known as 'mixed incontinence'.

Medicines Associated with Urinary Incontinence

Medicines can also exacerbate urinary incontinence, so it is good to be aware of them. Some of these medicines are:

- alpha-adrenergic agonists – may be used to treat hypotension or bradycardia
- alpha-adrenergic blockers – may be used to treat hypertension or erectile dysfunction
- angiotensin-converting enzymes – may be used to treat heart and kidney conditions
- diuretics – drugs used to increase diuresis
- cholinesterase inhibitors – may be used in the treatment of Alzheimer's disease
- some medications with anticholinergic effect – may be used in the treatment of Parkinson's disease
- hormone replacement therapy
- opioids
- sedatives
- hypnotics.

Table 4.2 Types of urinary incontinence.

Type of urinary incontinence	Presentation	Possible causes
Stress	Slight leakage of urine during any physical activity (sneezing, coughing, jogging, laughing) due to a rise in abdominal pressure.	Pregnancy, childbirth, estrogen withdrawal in menopause, obesity, pelvic-floor weakness, prostatic surgery
Urgency/urge	An involuntary loss of urine, accompanied by a strong desire to void.	Detrusor muscle instability, central nervous system problems, e.g. stroke (cerebrovascular accident), Parkinson's disease, multiple sclerosis, bladder, brain tumour, urinary tract infection, long-term indwelling catheter
Overflow	Involuntary, unpredictable loss of urine in the presence of a residual amount of urine in the bladder. Causes a stream of urine, leading to constant dampness, or may need to strain to void.	Sensory peripheral neuropathy (diabetic), spina bifida, Parkinson's disease, faecal impaction, urethral strictures, lower sacral cord injury, some anti-depressants
Reflex	Involuntary loss of urine when certain bladder volume is reached	Cerebrovascular accident, dementia, confusion, spinal injury above the level of S2, spina bifida
Environmental/ locomotor	Leakage of urine due to inability to toilet themselves	Cognitive impairment, confusion, physical disabilities

Promoting Continence

Containment

In relation to incontinence, containment is when an individual may be required to wear incontinence pads in the short or long term. These pads should never be stored in the bathroom, or any other warm, moist area, as they contain a silicone layer, which expands when moist. Incorrect storage will render these pads less effective.

The following are some of the areas that may need to be addressed when an individual is experiencing urinary incontinence:

- **Pelvic-floor exercises:** to strengthen this muscle set.
- **Bladder retraining:** to establish a regular pattern; keeping a bladder diary.
- **Adequate toileting:** the individual may require assistance to toilet and we may consider aids such as commodes, bedpans and urinals. Always remember to put them within easy reach.
- **Treat underlying disorders:** avoid constipation and assess for urinary tract infections by obtaining a urine sample and performing an urinalysis.
- **Adequate fluid intake:** the individual is encouraged to drink adequate fluids and to review fluid types, including bladder irritants such as coffee and cola (caffeine-based beverages).
- **Drug therapy:** a general practitioner (GP) may review present medications, such as sedatives.
- **Surgery:** a GP may refer the person to a continence advisor or urologist.
- **Improve environment:** the patient may find it difficult to mobilise to an upstairs toilet. We would need to conduct an assessment to find other factors that may be contributing to the incontinence (e.g. eyesight tests).
- **Containment:** pads or appliances.
- **Urinary drainage:** the individual may require urinary catheterisation, either intermittent or indwelling.

We must always report any concerns we have with service users, patients or any individual in our care to a nurse in charge, GP or member of the multidisciplinary team caring for the individual.

There are two main types of incontinence pad:

1. Shaped product used in conjunction with a fitting product (e.g. net pants).
2. All-in-one pad (Figure 4.2).

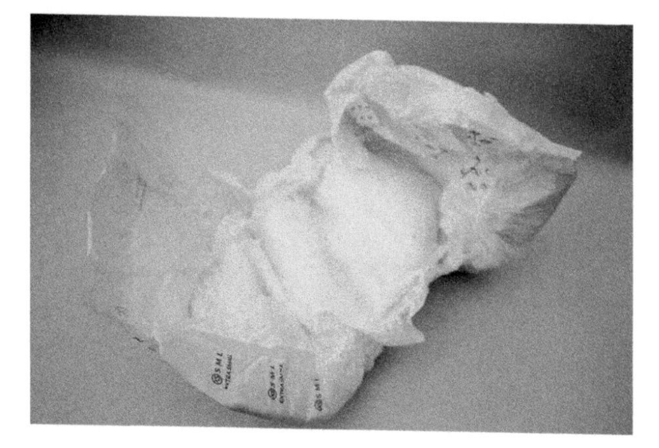

Figure 4.2 Incontinence pad.

The correct fitting of these pads is very important. These general rules apply:

- Do not touch the inside of the pad.
- The pad should fit neatly into the individual's groin.
- The back of the pad should be turned away from the body and groin.
- Apply the pad from the front to back and always remove the pad from behind.
- Do not use any talcum powder or oil-based barrier creams (which tend to block the pad's top dry layer).
- If an individual's skin is not marked or red, do not apply cream.
- The pad should be changed every three to four hours during the day and evening.
- The pad can be used for up to eight hours during the night to promote adequate sleep patterns.
- Do not store pads in a bathroom (damp environment) but in dry, warm surroundings.

Males

Men can also use a device called a penile clamp, which is exactly as it sounds – a clamp to be worn on the tip of the penis foreskin if urinary 'dribbling' is a problem. These devices can only be worn for short periods. Figure 4.3 shows

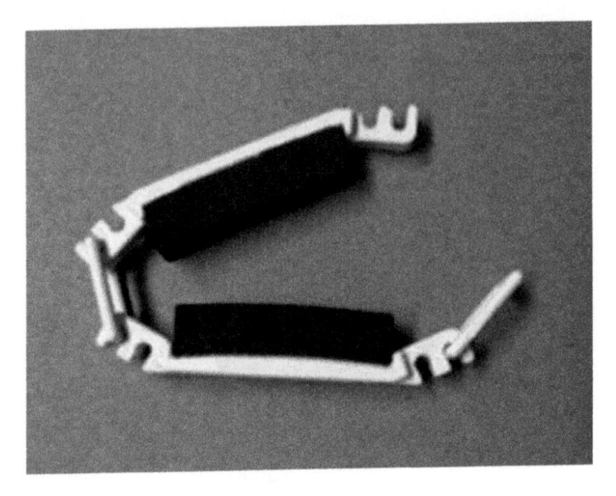

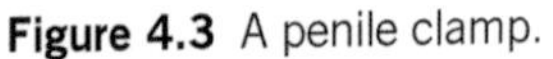

Figure 4.3 A penile clamp.

a penile clamp. When I used to show this device during my training sessions, all the men in the class would cross their legs!

Men also have the opportunity of the penile sheath (or convene), which is a much less invasive device than an indwelling catheter. The sheath is attached to a leg bag, which can be strapped to the leg enabling mobility.

FLUIDS

Encouraging a patient to drink more fluids is often called 'pushing fluids' in healthcare. We would also encourage drinking more caffeine-free drinks, and also the consumption of foods with a high water content, such as soup or ice cream. However, if an individual loves their cups of tea, and this is the only drink they will take, then we need to go with this, as it is individual choice. Remember: care and compassion.

FAECES

Faecal matter is composed of:

- 75% water
- 25% solid matter, comprising quantities of dead bacteria, fatty acids, inorganic matter, proteins, and undigested dietary fibre.

Faecal matter in the adult is normally brown in colour, soft and cylindrical. Faeces have an odour, due to the bacterial flora in the intestine, which varies according to the bacteria present and the food ingested.

The time it takes for undigested food to travel from the mouth through the alimentary canal and then out of the anus is known as the transit time, which is normally anything from one to three days in a young healthy adult. Older people may have an increased transit time of anything up to two weeks.

Babies and Children

Newborn babies excrete meconium waste matter from their bowels in an involuntary fashion. Meconium is a greenish-black sticky substance consisting of mucus, endothelial cells, amniotic fluid, bile pigments and fats.

After a few days the stools become a brownish-green in colour, then yellow.

Breastfed babies produce a softer, brighter yellow stool than bottle-fed infants, whose stools are paler and more formed. Once the child is weaned and eating a balanced diet the faeces become more like an adult's in composition.

Bowel Assessment

When conducting a full bowel assessment, components should be identified before any care package and treatments can commence:

- usual stool consistency
- usual stool frequency
- pain associated with bowel motion
- presence of blood and/or mucus
- evacuation problems
- past medical history
- toilet access issues
- diet and fluid intake
- medication, including over-the-counter medications.

Any changes in the normal bowel pattern could indicate bowel dysfunction.

Many healthcare areas use the Bristol Stool Chart, and you may wish to reacquaint yourself with this chart in Chapter 7, where we see that faeces with types 3 and 4 are suggested as the 'perfect poo'.

Bowel Dysfunction

It has been estimated that 1–10% of adults may experience some form of faecal incontinence. It is tolerated by carers to a lesser degree than urinary incontinence. For the person involved, faecal incontinence is an embarrassing and undignified condition, having a detrimental effect on one's psychological, social and physical wellbeing.

Causes of Bowel Dysfunction

Groups at high risk of faecal incontinence include:

- people with loose stools or diarrhoea from any cause
- women following childbirth (especially following third- or fourth-degree obstetric injury)
- people with neurological or spinal disease (e.g. spina bifida, stroke, multiple sclerosis or spinal cord injury)
- people with severe cognitive impairment
- people with urinary incontinence
- people with pelvic organ prolapse and/or rectal prolapse
- people who have had colonic resection or anal surgery
- people who have undergone pelvic radiotherapy
- people with perianal soreness, itching or pain
- people with learning disabilities.

After a cause has been established, a treatment plan can be initiated. Treatment options may include strengthening the pelvic floor muscles. Like all muscles in the body, the more they are used and exercised the stronger and firmer they will become.

Pelvic Floor Exercises

This pelvic floor exercise can be done sitting down or standing up. Ask the patient to imagine sitting on the toilet passing urine. Now they should imagine stopping the flow of urine, trying to really 'pull' upwards and squeeze and stop it.

This may be hard to start with. Some people can manage this upward movement in discrete stages, much like a lift going up past floors in a building! With practice, suggest that they try holding for a few seconds and then relaxing and letting go.

Ask the patient to sit down with the knees slightly apart. Tell them to imagine trying to stop themselves passing wind from the bowel. They should really squeeze and lift the muscle around the back passage. They should feel the skin around the back passage being pulled up and away from the chair and should feel the muscle move, but the buttocks and legs should not move.

These exercises can be done at any time, in any place, and no one need know! Tell the patient not to worry if they cannot feel the muscles very well; over time, the pelvic floor will strengthen and tighten and they will gain more control over it.

Another good exercise to strengthen the pelvic floor, as long as the patient does not have back, hip, or knee pain and discomfort, is the pelvic tilt, as follows.

Tell the patient to stand with feet 30 cm apart and knees slightly bent. Then ask them to rotate their hips in a clockwise circular movement for approximately 10 minutes. They should do this every day.

Other tips to firm up these muscles include avoiding high-impact exercises, which weaken the pelvic floor muscle. In contrast, yoga, pilates, swimming, cycling and belly dancing are considered good exercises for the pelvic floor. There are also exercise devices to be used to strengthen the pelvic floor (worn between the thighs) and electronic devices also on the market.

Moisture Lesions

We have seen that pelvic floor weakness can be a cause of incontinence, which may in turn cause moisture-induced skin damage if the urine and/or faeces (and even perspiration) is in continuous contact with the skin around such areas as:

- perineum
- buttocks

- groins
- inner thighs
- natal cleft
- skin folds
- where skin is in contact with skin (e.g. under the breasts).

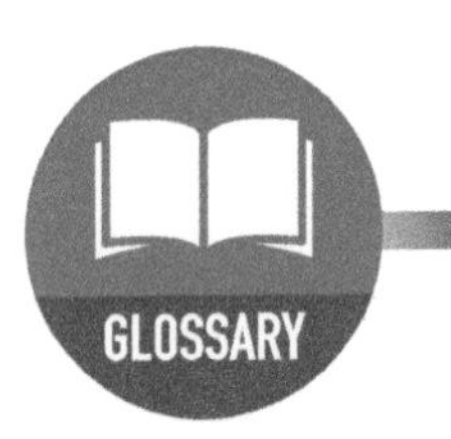

Perineum

The area between the anus and the scrotum (males) or vulva (females).

Natal cleft

The groove between the buttocks that runs from just below the sacrum to the perineum (also known as gluteal cleft or 'bottom crack').

Moisture lesions caused by incontinence are also known as 'incontinence-associated dermatitis' and in babies as 'nappy rash'. They can occur in any age group but in the older age group the skin is more fragile and can become damaged more easily. Prolonged exposure causes the skin to become more permeable, making the skin weaker and less elastic and more susceptible to physical damage from friction and shearing. Damaged skin can also lead to an increased risk of bacterial infection. Moisture lesions can also be very painful because they tend to be very shallow wounds with the nerve endings exposed. Not all moisture lesions are caused by urine and faeces.

There are four types of moisture-associated skin damage:

1. Incontinence-associated dermatitis (IAD) – where the ammonia from urine and enzymes from the stools disrupts the acid mantle of the skin (natural pH) causing the skin to break down.
2. Periwound moisture-associated dermatitis – where the leaky wound's enzymes cause maceration (moisture damage) of the surrounding skin of the wound.

3. Peristomal moisture-associated dermatitis – where inflammation and erosion of the skin related to the moisture spill from the stoma site.
4. Intertriginous dermatitis – where excessive sweating can lead to a build-up of moisture in the folds and creases of the skin, such as inguinal skin folds, axillary folds and under the breasts.

There is often confusion between pressure ulcers and moisture lesions. It is important to distinguish between the two, as treatment may differ. Table 4.3 shows the clinical presentation of moisture lesions and pressure ulcers.

Table 4.3 Clinical presentation of moisture lesions and pressure ulcers.

Characteristic	Moisture lesion	Pressure ulcer
Cause	Moisture must be present (e.g. urine, diarrhoea)	Pressure and/or shear must be present
Location	Perineum, buttocks, inner thigh, groin, skin folds, and may occur over bony prominence	Mainly occurs over bony prominence. May be equipment related (e.g. under a device/tube)
Shape	Diffuse differential areas/spots; kissing ulcer (e.g. under breasts); anal cleft – linear	Circular wounds, regular shape
Depth	Superficial partial thickness skin loss, but can enlarge if infection is present	Dependent on category of ulcer
Necrosis	No necrosis	Dependent on category of ulcer
Edge	Diffuse and irregular	Raised
Colour of the wound bed	Non-uniform redness; pink/white surrounding skin; perianal redness	Erythema, slough, necrosis, granulation tissue, epithelial tissue, dressing residue, infection
Distribution	Confluent (merging) patchy	Isolated individual lesions

ASSESSMENT

It is important to prevent moisture lesions from occurring. We do this through robust assessment of:

- skin
- continence
- nutrition
- falls and manual handling (as individuals may need assistance mobilising to the toilet).

PROTECTING THE SKIN AND MANAGING INCONTINENCE-ASSOCIATED DERMATITIS

To minimise the occurrence of moisture lesions caused by incontinence it is important to inform those involved that incontinence is not an inevitable consequence of old age and much can be done to manage it. One intervention is to protect the skin by keeping it clean and dry and by using:

- protective skin barriers
- gentle cleansers
- simple moisturisers
- incontinence products, such as incontinence pads
- faecal management systems.

Table 4.4 shows the best practice for managing IAD – the do's and don'ts.

Table 4.4 Dos and don'ts for the best practice of managing incontinence-associated dermatitis.

Do	**Establish the cause of the problem**
	To assess severity of the problem, record all episodes of incontinence
	Establish a skin care regimen with timely cleansing of soiled and wet skin

Table 4.4 (Continued)

	Use barrier products (films or creams) if the skin is reddened or broken to act as a barrier to prevent further damage
	Use incontinence products and faecal management systems to help avoid skin contact with urine and faeces
	To prevent pressure damage, smooth incontinence pads before use
	Inspect skin regularly (including night time if appropriate)
	Use foam cleaners when cleansing following episodes of incontinence
	Encourage good hydration, which will dilute the urine
	Identify incontinence and those with mobility issues who are at high risk of pressure ulcer development
	Seek advice from continence advisor/specialised nurse
Do NOT	Use traditional soap and water when cleansing following episodes of incontinence
	Use multiple incontinence pads
	Use creams and talcum powders under barrier products
	Assume that incontinence in the older person is inevitable

TEST YOUR KNOWLEDGE

1. What is enuresis?
2. What is night-time bed wetting called?
3. Name three types of urinary incontinence.
4. What is the stool of a newborn baby called?
5. What are the questions you should ask the service user or patient when conducting a thorough bowel assessment?
6. Faecal matter is composed of what two things?
7. What is another name for the natal cleft?
8. What is IAD?
9. What is the difference between a moisture lesion and a pressure ulcer's wound edge?
10. What four assessments should be conducted to minimise the prevalence of moisture lesions?

KEY POINTS

- The composition of urine and specific gravity.
- Types and causes of urinary incontinence.
- Promoting continence.
- The composition of faeces.
- Causes of bowel dysfunction.
- Moisture lesions.

USEFUL WEB RESOURCES

Bladder and Bowel Foundation: www.bladderandbowelfoundation.org

Brighton and Sussex University Hospitals NHS Trust. *Moisture Lesions and Incontinence Associated Dermatitis*. Information for patients and carers: https://www.bsuh.nhs.uk/documents/moisture-lesions-and-incontinence-associated-dermatitis

British Association of Urological Surgeons: www.baus.org.uk

NHS. Overview: Urinary incontinence: www.nhs.uk/conditions/urinary-incontinence

NHS. Squeezy app. Pelvic floor exercises for men and women: www.squeezyapp.com

Chapter 5

MALE URETHRAL CATHETERISATION

LEARNING OUTCOMES

By the end of this chapter you will have an understanding of the theory and practice of performing the clinical skill of male urethral catheterisation.

Urinary catheterisation can be defined as 'the insertion of a special tube into the bladder, using aseptic technique, for the purpose of *evacuating* or *instilling* fluids'.

DID YOU KNOW?

Catheters can be inserted when a patient requires a 'bladder wash out' if they have clots or debris etc. in the bladder. But many healthcare workers still think that urinary catheters are only inserted for drainage.

Catheters are hollow tubes with an eyelet at one end (which sits in the bladder) to facilitate drainage of urine along and out of the tube. Indwelling urethral catheters have a balloon to hold the tube in place in the bladder (Figure 5.1).

Catheters are measured in Charrières (abbreviated to Ch), which is the circumference of the catheter in millimetres, equivalent to three times the diameter. Therefore a 12 Ch catheter has a diameter of 4 mm. Most adult male urethral catheterisations are performed using a 12 Ch or a 14 Ch catheter. The scale is also called the French scale, abbreviated to Fr gauge.

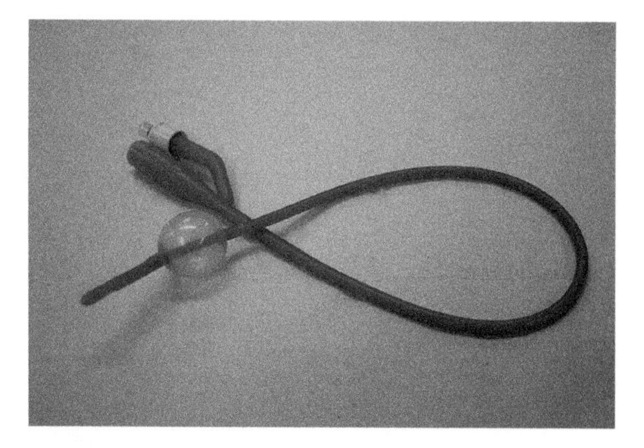

Figure 5.1 Indwelling urethral catheter, with balloon inflated.

POLICIES AND PROCEDURES

When performing the clinical procedure of urinary catheterisation, your own employer's policy should be read and cross-referenced to other policies in your area, such as those on:

- universal infection-control precautions
- hand hygiene
- disposal of waste
- handling and transportation of pathology specimens policy
- collection and transport of clinical specimens
- consent: assessment of mental capacity and determining best interests (documented)
- use of latex
- chaperones.

Reading these policies and procedures is to protect the patient, and you, to ensure that you do not break 'vicarious liability', which can be defined as the principle by which a practitioner's employer will take liability for the actions and omissions of the employee as long as they are acting within their job description and boundaries approved by the employer.

In short, we must follow the safety measures (i.e. the policies and procedures) that have been put in place, and act within our job description and our employer's boundaries.

WHY IS URINARY CATHETERISATION PERFORMED?

Prior to undertaking urethral catheterisation, we need to conduct a thorough assessment of our patient. Usually, urinary catheterisation is undertaken under three main categories: for drainage, for investigation or for instillation.

Drainage

- Bladder outflow obstruction.
- Acute or chronic retention.
- Detrusor underactivity.
- Pre- and post-pelvic surgery (e.g. lower urinary tract surgery).
- Accurate measurement of urine output.
- Determination of residual volume.
- Comfort for the terminally ill.
- Prevention of skin breakdown.
- Relief of incontinence when no other means is practicable.

Investigation

- To obtain an uncontaminated urine specimen if one is unobtainable by non-invasive methods.
- In urodynamic investigations.
- X-ray investigations.

Instillation

- To irrigate the bladder.
- To instil medication (e.g. chemotherapy).

The assessment should also consider:

- cognitive status
- the patient's ability to manage the catheter, if appropriate
- carer availability to support catheter care, if appropriate
- tissue viability and preservation of skin integrity.

If a patient lacks the mental capacity to consent to the procedure, it may still be carried out in their best interests and documented accordingly.

FLUID OUTPUT

When I first did my nurse training, we talked constantly about meeting the '30ml per hour' target, as we thought this was the magic figure for urine output that all patients needed to achieve for us to know that their renal function was not impaired. We now know this is not true: a 107kg man will not have the same output as a 50kg older woman! What were we thinking? Thank goodness for evidence-based nursing! Let me show you what this means in practice.

But even using the formula does not give us the whole picture, as medical conditions such as hypotension may mean that the kidneys are not being fully perfused. This patient may have a congested cardiac condition and may be prescribed a diuretic medication such as furosemide. Many patients call these pills 'water tablets' as they cause increased micturition. This woman may be critically ill and experiencing 'peripheral shutdown' or may become dehydrated. In short, we need to look at the patient holistically: this means looking at the whole picture and not using a formula like the one given above in isolation.

e.g.
EXAMPLE

Let me show you an example. . .

Using the old system, we'd expect a 70 kg person to produce 30 ml of urine each hour. In 24 hours, this equates to 720 ml (30 ml × 24 hours = 720 ml). This does not take into account the person's body weight, however.

Now, if we use the formula:

$$\text{urine output} = 0.5\,\text{ml}/\text{kg}/\text{hour}$$

This does take into account the person's body weight. So, for a 70 kg woman, inputting this body weight into the formula, we find that daily urine output would be expected to be:

$$0.5\text{ml} \times 70\text{kg} \times 24\text{hours} = 840$$

This makes a huge difference: 120 ml. Putting this into practice, we thought that 720 ml was satisfactory when in effect this output was too low, as a person of this size should be producing 840 ml every day.

HIGH-RISK PROCEDURE

Urinary catheterisation is classed as a high-risk procedure, as it is very often the mode for micro-organisms to enter the human body.

Many trusts have adapted the Saving Lives tools to collect data on infections in these core areas and report their infection rates to the Department of Health. Trusts then incur fines if the numbers are higher than they should be. In the case of urinary catheter care, there is a weekly audit of every patient in the clinical area with a urinary catheter in place, and infections are reported. So, although the campaign has now officially been completed, the infection rates audit is still being maintained.

DID YOU KNOW?

Historical Facts

In the first part of this century, The UK Department of Health instigated the Saving Lives campaign, which was a delivery programme to reduce healthcare-associated infections such as methicillin-resistant *Staphylococcus aureus* (MRSA) and included reducing the incidence of urinary tract infections (UTIs). The programme provided tools for acute trusts to make significant reductions to infection rates of MRSA bloodstream infections by 2008. The high impact areas were:

- High impact intervention no. 1: preventing the risk of microbial contamination
- High impact intervention no. 2: central venous catheter care
- High impact intervention no. 3: preventing surgical site infection
- High impact intervention no. 4: care of ventilated patients
- High impact intervention no. 5: urinary catheter care.

When we catheterise a patient in an NHS hospital, we need to collect data and report every incidence of catheter-associated UTI (or CAUTI). Urinary catheterisation is high impact intervention no. 5, due to it being reported that:

- more than 40% of all hospital-acquired infections are CAUTIs
- there is a daily risk rate of 5–8% of developing a CAUTI
- 20–30% of catheterised patients develop bacteriuria; 2–6% of these develop UTIs
- 4% of these patients develop bacteraemia and 13–30% of them die
- 80% of all CAUTIs are caused on insertion.

Male catheterisation has always been considered as an 'advanced role' separate from female catheterisation. This is because males have a prostate gland, which could potentially be punctured during the process of inserting the catheter.

As men head towards their 'three score years and ten' (that is, age 70), the prostate naturally enlarges. This is a very vascular process, meaning that if the gland does get punctured the patient could bleed to death.

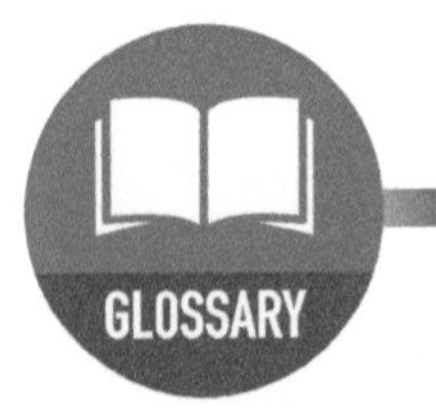

Vascular
Relating to or supplied with blood.

PERSONAL CARE AND THE NEED FOR STRICT ASEPSIS

As a catheter tube is a 'foreign body' within the body, we need to take particular care with the patient's personal care, so as not to introduce microbes into their system. One of the entry points for these microbes is the join between the catheter tube and the attached drainage bag. It is for this reason that the connection between the catheter and the urinary drainage system must not be broken, except when renewing the catheter bag.

Practitioners must also decontaminate their hands using the six-step handwash technique with water and soap or alcohol gel, and must wear non-sterile gloves before manipulation of the catheter system.

Meatal and suprapubic site care must be carried out with unperfumed soap and water daily, or as required if build-up of secretions is evident. I can't tell you the number of times I have pulled back a foreskin and found a substance akin to cream cheese! This is due to a build-up of the bacteria that we do not want to travel up the catheter tubing into the bladder, to cause a systemic catheter-associated infection.

Perfumed soap may cause irritation to this sensitive area. Remember, not all men have a foreskin; for those with a foreskin, it should be eased down gently over the catheter after cleaning, in order not to cause a paraphimosis.

Talcum powder and creams should not be used around catheter sites, as they may cause microbe colonisation by travelling up the catheter tube. As we wipe the catheter tubing, we wipe away from the body, down the tube.

The drainage bag should be positioned above the floor but below bladder level to prevent reflux or contamination. Obviously, this is not the case with 'belly bags', which are worn around the waist. All drainage bags should be hung either on a catheter stand or a bed-hanger stand. They should never be dragged along on the floor, as this will cause the bag to pick up germs.

During catheter insertion, strict asepsis must be maintained. Dressing packs for this procedure come in many different varieties. Check to see if your pack contains sterile gloves or whether you will need to put a pack on to your dressing trolley.

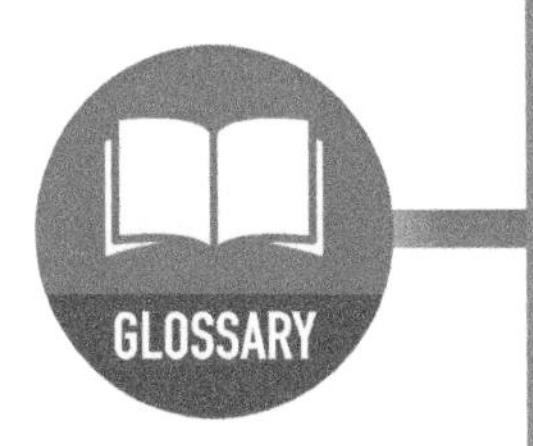

Paraphimosis

A paraphimosis is a tightening of the foreskin behind the glans penis. The foreskin is unable to be drawn back, causing pain and swelling to the penis, and may need surgery to rectify. When bladder hyper-irritability occurs, a medic may prescribe diazepam to stop the urethra going into spasm. The carer may also need to consider inserting a smaller catheter of different material, as this may be causing the irritability to the urethra and leakage of urine to occur.

ANATOMY AND PHYSIOLOGY

Before we can begin to learn a new clinical skill, we need to have some knowledge of the basic anatomy and physiology associated with the skill.

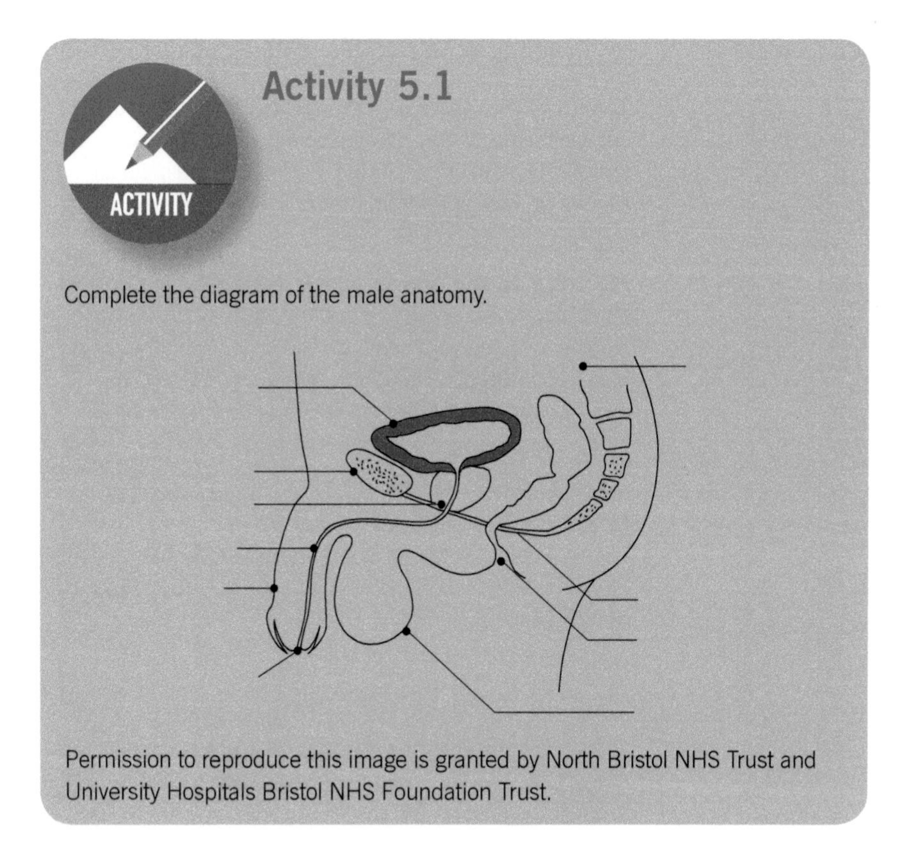

Activity 5.1

Complete the diagram of the male anatomy.

Permission to reproduce this image is granted by North Bristol NHS Trust and University Hospitals Bristol NHS Foundation Trust.

The main function of the kidneys is to act as a filtration system and to maintain bodily fluid, electrolyte and acid–base balance. These organs also play a part in synthesis of vitamin D and the detoxification of free radicals and drugs.

The ureters are tubular organs than run from the renal pelvis to the bladder. They are approximately 25–30cm in length and 5mm in diameter in adults. Their purpose is to transport urine from the renal pelvis into the bladder.

The bladder is a hollow muscular organ that stores urine. It is usually able to hold between 350 and 750 ml of urine in adults. In the inner floor of the bladder is the nerve supply, or trigone. These sensory nerves travel to the brain and pass on signals that the bladder requires emptying. Motor nerves are then activated to inform the detrusor muscle, and internal and external sphincters to allow urine to flow out from the bladder along the urethra.

In males, the urethra is approximately 15–20 cm in length. It has to pass through the prostate gland before reaching the penis. The prostate is a vascular organ that produces fluid that forms part of the semen.

The Prostate

Tests to determine an enlarged prostate usually take the form of a digital examination, whereby two gloved and lubricated fingers are inserted up the man's anus to feel for the prostate. The prostate should be walnut-sized, relatively soft and slightly spongy.

A screen for prostate-specific antigens (PSA) can also be done, in the form of a simple blood test. However, although these tests are becoming more accurate, they may give a false positive if the patient has been massaging his scrotum, has recently had sexual intercourse and/or has recently had a rectal examination, all of which cause a rise in PSA levels.

The definitive test in the UK for prostate malignancy is currently a biopsy. Research by the Institute of Cancer Research UK has looked at the link between male finger length and the risk of developing prostate cancer (Rahman et al. 2010). The finding is that those with longer ring fingers are more at risk. Here's how to assess this:

1. Measure from the crease at the bottom of the ring finger to the tip (this is the finger next to the little finger).
2. Measure from the crease at the bottom of the index finger to the tip (this is the finger next to the thumb).
3. Men with longer index fingers than ring fingers are significantly less likely to get prostate cancer.

It is all to do with the amount of the hormone testosterone that a baby is exposed to in the womb. Being exposed to less testosterone equates to a longer index finger and a reduced chance of getting prostate cancer in later life.

CATHETERISATION

There are three types of urinary catheterisation.

1. *Intermittent:* the lubricated catheter tube is inserted into the bladder, up the urethra, to drain urine every four to six hours. The tube is withdrawn each time and disposed of. A clean technique is performed. Patients performing this procedure on themselves are taught how to do it. It does require willpower, dexterity and good cognitive function. This method of catheterisation can give individuals independence and control over their own bodies. It used to be called intermittent 'self-catheterisation' but as many carers now perform the technique it is now commonly known as clean intermittent catheterisation (or CIC).
2. *Urethral:* here, the catheter is inserted up the urethra and a balloon is gently blown up at the bladder end with approximately 10 ml of water (or however much water is required for a particular catheter). The catheter is then secured in place. Urethral catheters can be left in place over the longer term (days or months), and consequently have higher incidences of infection. At the end of the catheter tubing, a drainage bag needs to be in place to collect the urine. Some individuals may not wish to use a drainage bag but instead have a valve, which works like a tap to drain the urine from the bladder, along the catheter tubing and out through the valve. It is not certain why indwelling catheterisation began to be used more frequently than self-catheterisation, but an advantage of this method of catheterisation is that it can be used over the course of long surgical procedures and when individuals are having bed rest, if deemed appropriate. This is also known as indwelling urethral catheterisation, as the catheter remains in place.

3. *Suprapubic:* this is where the catheter is inserted through the anterior abdominal wall into bladder, whereby a stoma is created. A dressing is initially applied around the stoma but can be removed after three to five days, as warmth creates a higher incidence of infection. The wound should be observed for infection and overgranulation. An advantage of this method of catheterisation is that it can be used if urethral catheterisation is not feasible due to trauma, for example. In addition, suprapubic catheterisation (SPC) leaves the individual's genitals free for sexual activity. This is also known as indwelling SPC, as the catheter remains in place.

EXCLUSION CRITERIA FOR URETHRAL CATHETERISATION

Only specialist healthcare personnel should undertake urinary catheterisation on the following categories of individuals:

- within 48 hours of prostate surgery
- those who have a history of urethral stricture
- patients with a history of bacteraemia associated with catheterisation (unless the patient has been given appropriate antibiotic prophylaxis)
- those with symptomatic UTI (unless the patient has adequate antibiotic cover)
- patients with a priapism.

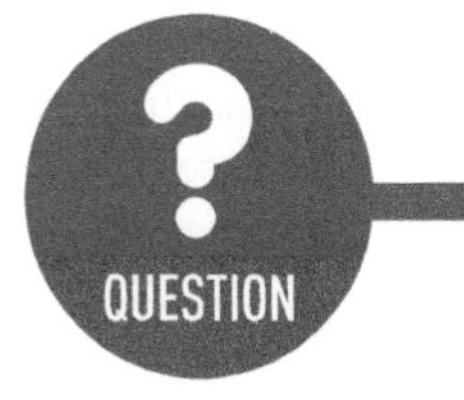

Question 5.1 What is a urethral stricture?
Question 5.2 What is a priapism?

CATHETER MATERIAL AND SELECTION

Indwelling urethral catheters came in a variety of materials and designs, depending on the rationale for insertion and insertion time. A balloon is inflated to keep the catheter in place in the bladder. A rule of thumb is that the smallest-possible catheter should be chosen to maintain drainage.

Catheters are usually categorised in one of three time scales, depending on how long the catheter is expected to be in place, with the catheter material reflecting this:

short term (1–14 days)
short to medium term (two to six weeks)
medium to long term (six weeks to three months).

- PTFE (polytetrafluoroethylene)/silver-coated catheters: these are usually inserted for up to 28 days. They are soft, but this allows crust formation. Teflon-coated or silicone (PTFE) elastomer-coated catheters have a latex core. This reduces urethral irritation. Silver-alloy coated catheters are thought to reduce bacterial colonisation in the longer term.
- Hydrogel-coated latex catheters: these are used for up to 12 weeks. They are well tolerated by the urethral mucosa, causing little irritation to the mucosal lining. They are reported to be resistant to bacterial colonisation and encrustation.
- All-silicone catheters: these are used for up to 12 weeks. They have a wider lumen, which is crescent or D-shaped but as they are rigid, they may be more uncomfortable. They are the only sort suitable for patients with a latex allergy.
- Hydrophilic catheters: these are for intermittent use. They are lubricated for ease of insertion, and come in a variety of designs. Figure 5.2 shows a selection of these catheters.

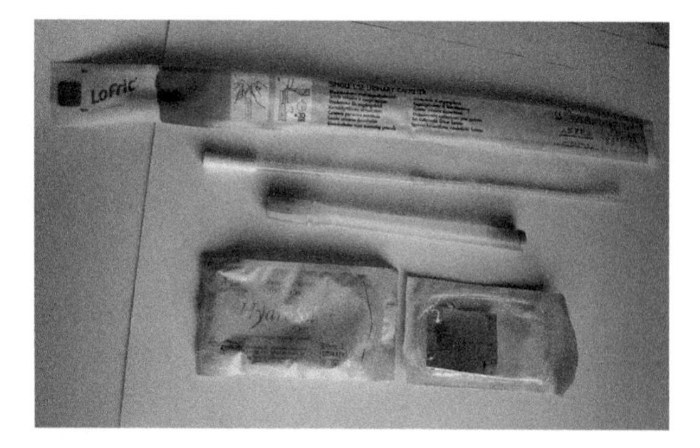

Figure 5.2 A selection of intermittent catheters.

Whichever catheter is selected, all catheters should be stored flat in their original boxes and in a cool place. They should never be stored tied with rubber bands as this can bend the catheter and distort the water channel.

CATHETER LENGTH AND DESIGN

Catheters come in three lengths:

- standard (or 'male' length), 40–44 cm
- female length, 23–26 cm
- paediatric length, 30 cm.

Figure 5.3 shows a standard-length and a female-length catheter.

The UK National Patient Safety Agency (NPSA; a Department of Health watchdog until 2012) issued an alert stating the dangers of inserting a shorter, female-length catheter into a male and the damage that it could cause when the balloon is inflated in the urethra rather than the bladder. The NPSA reported that in one 12-month period there were 114 incidents where female catheters were inserted into male patients. All experienced severe pain, some degree of

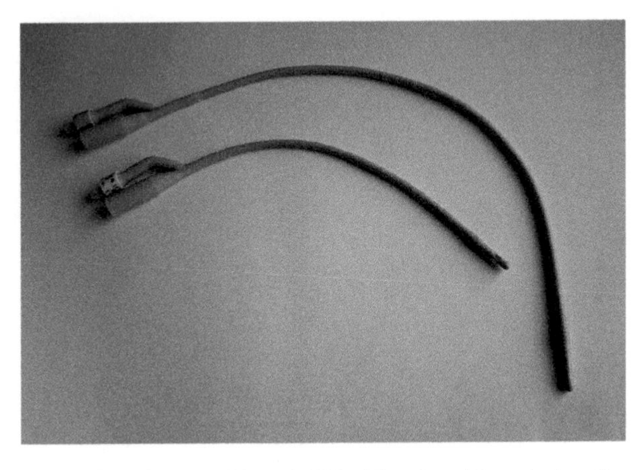

Figure 5.3 Standard-length (40–44 cm) and female-length (23–26 cm) catheters. Note that in many care settings only standard-length catheters are now used.

haematuria, penile swelling or retention. Seven of these insertions caused significant haemorrhage, with two believed to have led to acute renal failure, and two to impaired renal function. It was due to this alert that many care settings removed the shorter-length catheters and now only insert the standard length into all patients (male and female).

> Adult urinary catheters are manufactured in two lengths: female length (20–26 cm), and standard length (40–45 cm). The use of standard length catheters in females poses no safety issues, as the shorter female length is designed for dignity issues when wearing skirts rather than trousers. However, if a female length catheter is accidentally used for a male, the 'balloon' inflated with sterile water to retain the catheter will be within the urethra, rather than the bladder, and can then cause severe trauma
>
> (National Patient Safety Agency 2009).

Since this safety alert, we have all become more aware of catheter lengths.

Catheters are also available in designs other than with the standard round tip. This is to resolve particular problems associated with urinary catheterisation. For example, a Tieman-tipped catheter has a curved tip with up to three drainage eyes for greater drainage. Some patients may experience an output of urine with large amounts of debris and/or clots, so a larger catheter with larger eyelets or multiple eyelets may be used.

REMOVING THE CATHETER

There must be a daily review of the need for the catheter with a view to removing it as soon as possible.

Catheters should be removed following assessment of the individual's continuing condition and in consultation with the individual and the multidisciplinary team responsible for their care. The balloon will need to be deflated to allow the catheter tube to be pulled out through the urethra. The balloon valve must never be cut off. If difficulty is experienced during the process of deflation, assistance must be sought immediately.

When deflating the balloon to remove the catheter, just attach a syringe to the balloon valve on the catheter tube and allow the balloon to self-drain. *Do not aspirate* (i.e. draw back) the syringe as this pulls the mucosal wall into the catheter eyelet and may cause damage. With silicone catheters, the balloon takes longer to drain, so you do need to be patient, but it only takes only a matter of moments in most cases. The longer the catheter has been in place, the longer the balloon will take to deflate.

After removal, fluid intake and output must be monitored carefully to ensure the bladder is emptying efficiently and that there are no episodes of incontinence.

DRAINAGE BAGS AND SECURING DEVICES

As the urine flows from the catheter tubing, a drainage device needs to be attached. These devices come in a variety of designs, such as leg bags for ambulatory patients, where the bag is attached to the patient's leg.

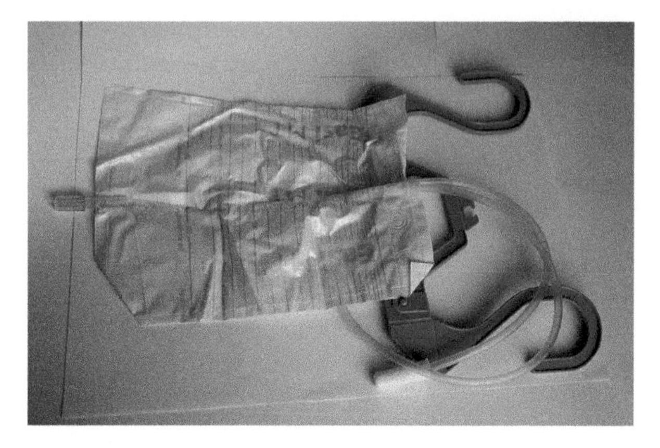

Figure 5.4 A night bag attached to a frame.

At night, a 'night bag' can be attached to a leg bag or other drainage day bag to collect larger volumes of urine (Figure 5.4). Night bags can be attached to a frame and these may be further attached to the bed frame. In the morning, the night bag is detached, leaving the leg or day bag in place. Always remember to close the tap first before detaching the night bag, otherwise the urine will pour all over your shoes!

When emptying these bags, a closed system must be maintained, so as not to expose the patient to microbial contamination.

Some individuals prefer to use a waist 'belly bag', which is actually just as the name suggests: it is worn around the waist, much like a 'bum bag'. It works on the principle of venous pressure pushing the urine upwards into the waist bag. Figure 5.5 shows one of these systems.

Leg bags are usually changed every 5–7 days and belly bags every 28 days.

Whichever drainage bag has been selected, bags should be stabilised and secured (Figure 5.6). This is to prevent movement and pulling of the catheter tube, which in turn may cause trauma. Stabilisation may be maintained with the use of T-straps, aqua-sleeves or Statlock® (Bard) Foley stabilisation devices. A Statlock stabilisation device is a strap-free device that locks a Foley catheter in place.

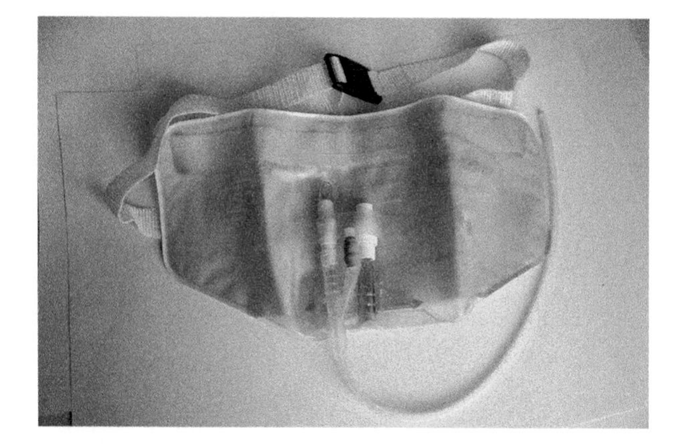

Figure 5.5 A catheter waist drainage bag.

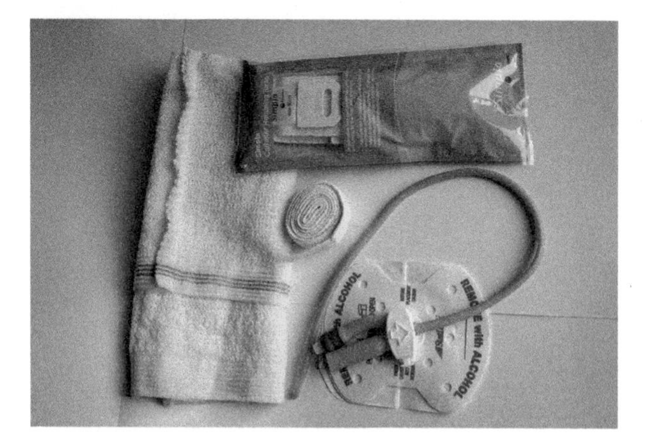

Figure 5.6 Catheter stabilisation devices.

The device is attached to the inner leg, much like a plaster, and is changed every seven days.

Patients, often in acute care, may require a UnoMeter® (Uno Medical), which is a diuresis-measuring system whereby acute urine output measures can be obtained.

Some individuals may prefer to use a catheter valve, which mimics normal bladder function (Figure 5.7). This is a valve that the individual opens intermittently to drain the bladder and which eliminates the need for a drainage bag. A valve usually gets replaced after seven days.

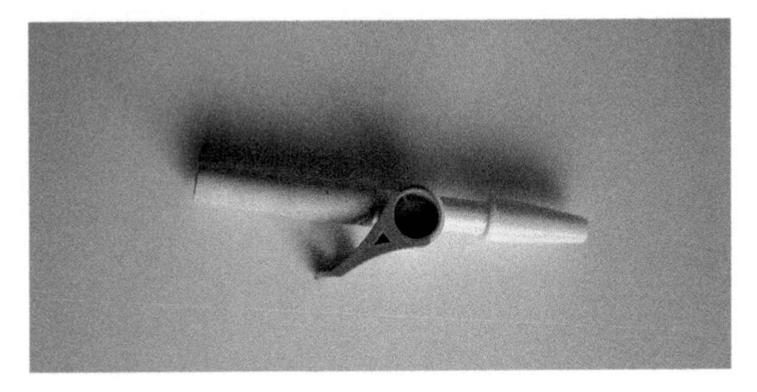

Figure 5.7 A catheter valve device.

Latex

Only latex-free catheters can be inserted into individuals with latex sensitivity, otherwise they could experience a full-blown allergic reaction causing anaphylaxis. Individuals known to have a sensitivity to certain foodstuffs, such as kiwi fruit, avocados and bananas, will also need to avoid anything containing latex, as these foods contain the same proteins as latex and could cause a reaction.

Latex-sensitive patients will also need to receive their care with latex-free gloves, to avoid a reaction.

Lubrication

Much has been written on the subject of the lubrication to be used when inserting the catheter. Many areas use lignocaine-based lubricants, with anaesthetic properties. If these substances are used, they must be left to work for approximately five minutes before the catherization can take place. However, there are contraindications to these products, especially in patients with certain cardiac arrhythmias, hypertension, hepatic problems and epilepsy and so on, so many areas have gone back to using water-based lubrication, such as KY® Jelly. It is important to find out the practice in your area. It is important to also note that lubrication *must* be used for both males and females (not just males as some medics informed me).

Antibiotic Cover

Again, much has been written about the use of prophylactic antibiotics in routine catheterisation. The use of antibiotics in these circumstances has not been supported by evidence-based research, and, indeed, the high incidence of increased resistance to antibiotics has been attributed to their overuse in the past. Some areas ask those prescribing antibiotics for routine catheterisations to consult a microbiologist to see if it is warranted. As nurses, we may be the ones expected to administer this antibiotic, either orally or by injection, so it is important to check the rationale for the prescription.

PROBLEMS ASSOCIATED WITH CATHETERISATION

The act of inserting a urethral catheter may present many complications to the patient, immediately and over the duration of its placement. Some of these problems may include:

- urethral trauma resulting in infection and possible septicaemia/renal failure/death
- formation of false urethral passage
- bladder perforation
- traumatic removal of catheter with balloon inflated
- urinary tract infection and possible septicaemia/renal failure/death
- bypassing of urine around catheter
- urethral stricture formation
- meatal tears
- encrustation and bladder calculi
- urethral perforation
- pain
- bleeding
- bladder spasm

- reduced bladder capacity
- catheter blockage
- latex sensitivity
- altered body image
- difficulties with sexual relations.

One of the main considerations associated with urinary catheterisation is infection. Ninety per cent of catheterised individuals will get a UTI within four weeks of a urethral catheterisation.

Other problems associated with catheterisation are:

- CAUTI
- tissue damage
- pressure necrosis
- abscess formation
- discomfort
- loss of dignity
- paraphimosis.

Good documentation must be performed when providing any clinical skill. In the case of catheterisation, certain information needs to be documented, such as:

- catheter type, length and size
- batch number
- manufacturer
- amount of water instilled into the balloon
- date and time of catheterisation
- reasons for catheterisation
- colour of urine drained
- any problems negotiated during the procedure
- a review date to assess the need for continued catheterisation or date of change of catheter.

If no urine drains, medical staff should be informed immediately. Continuing care is mediated by use of a catheter care plan, an example of which can be viewed in Figure 5.8.

Urinary Catheter Care Plan

North Bristol NHS

Indication for catheter?

- ☐ Accurate fluid balance (critically ill?)
- ☐ Urine retention
- ☐ Major Surgery
- ☐ Other (please specify):
- ☐ Urinary tract haemorrhage
- ☐ Palliative
- ☐ Skin breakdown from incontinence

Date of insertion: ....

Estimated date for removal or change: ....

Please record actions each shift.
Please record in boxes below ✓ =yes × =no
Please record A/C for actions that are daily or weekly and have already been completed
Please initial after each review at the bottom of the care plan

	Date																					
	Action	E	L	N	E	L	N	E	L	N	E	L	N	E	L	N	E	L	N	E	L	N
1.	**Hand hygiene** Before and after each patient contact																					
2.	**Catheter hygiene** Clean catheter site at least once a day as per policy CP1e																					
3.	**Drainage bag position** Above floor but below bladder level to prevent reflux or contamination and assist drainage																					
4.	**Sampling (needle-free) aseptically via catheter port**																					
5.	**Manipulation -Securing the catheter** Catheter secured using a fixation device using aseptic technique and comfortable for patient. Leg straps must be removed at night.																					
6.	**Manipulation - Catheter drainage bag emptying** Empty at least twice daily. Gloves and apron must be worn. Clean container used every time. Decontaminate port before emptying. Avoid touching drainage tap. Decontaminate hands after taking gloves and apron off.																					
7.	**Manipulation - Changing drainage bag** Urine drainage bags and valves must be dated and changed at least every 7 days.																					
8.	**Catheter needed?** Review daily, remove as soon as possible																					
	Please initial after each shift																					

SES. 22.12.10

Figure 5.8 *(Continued)*

Date	Variance	Sign

Guidance

Hand hygiene 5 moments
Before touching patient
Before clean. aseptic technique
After body fluid exposure
After touching patient
After touching patient surroundings

Sampling
Perform aseptically via the catheter port
Catheter manipulation (any action which involves touching the catheter system)
Examination gloves must be worn to manipulate a catheter, and manipulation should be preceded and followed by hand decontamination.
Maintain a closed system
Connection between catheter and drainage bag must not be broken except for good clinical reason e.g. changing drainage bag.
Single use non-drainable night bag may be used at night.
Recording
Record urinary output on fluid chart .if appropriate
Encourage good fluid intake.
Report poor output, (adequate output is 0.5 ml per kg of patient's body weight per hour e.g.33 mls if patient weighs 66 kgs.)
Report any changes in colour e.g. blood
Self management of hygiene & emptying
Following education and help if appropriate.
After removal of catheter
Ensure patient is within easy reach of a toilet or voiding receptacle.
Monitor intake and output, ensure patient is comfortable and feels that the bladder is empty after voiding.
Record episodes of incontinence.

For further information refer to: Policy for Adult Urethral Catheterisation and Supra-pubic Re-catheterisation Policy CP 1e

SES. 22.12.10

Figure 5.8 A urinary catheter care plan. Source: Reproduced with permission from North Bristol NHS Trust and University Hospitals Bristol NHS Foundation Trust.

HOW TO TAKE A CATHETER SAMPLE OF URINE

A catheter sample of urine is abbreviated to CSU. A CSU should only be taken:

- to diagnose UTI if the patient has systemic signs or symptoms consistent with a urinary infection
- as part of an MRSA screen when indicated
- for culture before elective orthopaedic implant surgery
- prior to defined urological procedures.

A CSU should not be taken just because:

- the urine is cloudy
- the urine in the bag is 'dipstick-positive', meaning that a urinalysis test has been performed and the urine contains elements that should not be present, such as protein, ketones, blood, sugar, etc.
- the catheter is blocked
- the urine smells offensive.

A sample of urine should always be obtained via the sample port and never via the drainage bag itself. The sample should be obtained under aseptic technique and after the sample port has been cleaned. Many sample ports are now designed for syringes only, known as 'needle-free sample ports'; these are usually red (Figure 5.9). Some areas may still use needle-and-syringe sample ports, which may be coloured blue. However, these are more prone to causing needlestick injuries. Both these ports 'self-seal' after the sample has been obtained.

EMPTYING A DRAINAGE BAG

An apron and gloves should be worn to empty a drainage bag. Prior to opening, the tap on the drainage device should be cleaned with an alcohol wipe (and again after the procedure). After the urine has been collected, the collection device should be covered when taking it to the sluice or toilet for disposal.

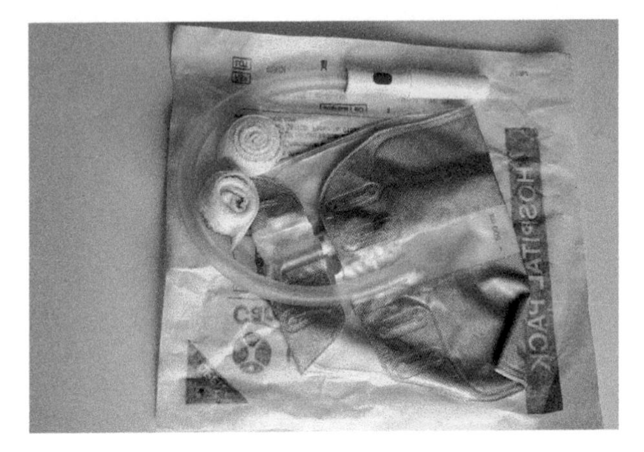

Figure 5.9 A needle-free sample port.

If the individual has a fluid chart, remember to measure the volume of urine and document it. Remove the apron and gloves and your wash hands with soap and water after each procedure.

How to empty a catheter drainage bag:

- Empty the drainage bag frequently enough to maintain urine flow and prevent reflux.
- Wash your hands.
- Use a clean pair of non-sterile gloves.
- Risk assess for need to wear face protection (goggles).
- Before emptying the bag, decontaminate the port with alcohol wipes.
- Urine bags should not be emptied into plastic reusable jugs, as this may cause cross-contamination.
- A separate and clean container should be used for each patient.
- Take care not to let the catheter drainage port the touch sides of the container.
- After emptying the catheter bag, the port should be decontaminated using alcohol wipes.

PROCEDURE FOR MALE URETHRAL CATHETERISATION

Now for the procedure of inserting the urethral catheter. Remember, it is usual to undertake this procedure after attending a study session and undergoing supervised practice before being deemed competent and confident to be able to perform the task. After the procedure, it is considered best practice to give the patient an information booklet or sheet that explains the procedure.

If the patient consents, have a 'runner' to hand; that is, someone who needs to learn the ropes and who can collect any equipment required during the procedure. For example, you may drop a piece of equipment and need to replace it. Never leave your patient exposed, even for a moment. In Chapter 6 we look at catheter all-in-one-boxes, whereby all the equipment is in one box.

Prior to catheterisation, the patient must have a good clean 'down below' with soap and water, so send them to the bathroom. Instruct them that, if they have a foreskin, they need to pull it back and wash underneath. Although we advocate self-care wherever possible, some patients may not be able to undertake this wash themselves, so we may need to take a bowl of warm water to the bedside and wash the patient ourselves. This wash is very important, as cleaning the meatus and penile shaft during the aseptic part with sodium chloride will not remove all the germs if the patient is very mucky down there.

The Equipment

- Sterile catheterisation pack.
- Disposable and waterproof pad.
- Sterile and non-sterile gloves.
- Appropriate size and length of catheter.
- Pre-packed sterile anaesthetic lubricating gel.
- Appropriate catheter valve and support accessories for catheter bag.
- Light source.

- Sterile water and syringe for the balloon (if not included in catheter pack).
- Disposable plastic apron.
- 1 drainage bag and stand or holder if appropriate.
- 0.9% sodium chloride (Normasol® sachet).
- Alcohol hand rub.
- Information leaflet/booklet with contact name if appropriate.

How to Catheterise a Male Patient

1. Explain and discuss the procedure with the patient. Gain consent.

2a. Screen the bed. Ensure good light source. Ask patient to shower or wash glans penis and scrotal area with soap and water in bathroom if able. Otherwise perform this task for the patient.

2b. Assist the patient to get into the semi-recumbent position with the legs extended.

2c. Do not expose the patient at this stage of the procedure. Ensure that the patient is warm.

3. Wash your hands using soap and water, using the six-step hand-washing technique.

4. Clean and prepare the trolley, placing all equipment required on the bottom shelf.

5. Take the trolley to the patient's bedside, disturbing screens as little as possible.

6. Open the outer cover of the catheterisation pack and slide the pack on to the top shelf of the trolley.

7. Using an aseptic technique, open the supplementary packs. Open catheter into sterile receiver.

8. Remove cover that is maintaining the patient's privacy and position a disposable pad under the patient's buttocks and thighs.

9. Put on a disposable plastic apron and non-sterile disposable gloves.

10. Retract the foreskin, if necessary, and clean the glans penis with 0.9% sodium chloride (Normasol), moving from the meatus to the base of the penis.

11. Remove non-sterile gloves and clean hands using the six-step technique with alcohol gel. Put on sterile gloves.
12. Place the sterile sheet with the hole over the penis.
13. Warn patient of the risk of stinging from the anaesthetic gel. Squeeze a drop of the single-use anaesthetic gel on to tip of catheter and also cover the meatus with gel. Then squeeze the remainder of the gel into urethra.
14. Hold the penis with a piece of gauze firmly for 3–5 minutes.
15. Hold the penis (at approximately 65 degrees) behind the glans, raising it until it is almost totally extended. Place the receiver containing the catheter between the patient's legs. Insert the catheter until urine flows and advance almost to the bifurcation.
16. If resistance is felt at the external sphincter, increase the traction on the penis slightly, and ask patient to cough and apply gentle, steady pressure on the catheter.
17. Gently inflate the balloon according to the manufacturer's instructions.
18. Withdraw the catheter slightly and attach it to a compatible valve or drainage system. Support the catheter by using a specifically designed support strap. Ensure that the catheter does not become taut when the patient mobilises.
19. Ensure that the glans penis is clean and reposition the foreskin.
20. Make the patient comfortable. Ensure that the area is dry.
21. If this is the first catheterisation, after 20 minutes, measure the amount of urine drained.
22. Dispose of equipment and gloves in a clinical waste bag and seal the bag before moving the trolley.
23. Draw back the curtains.
24. Dispose of clinical waste bag into a clinical waste bin.
25. Wash and dry hands thoroughly as per the six-step procedure and document all information.

TEST YOUR KNOWLEDGE

1. What are the three main methods of catheterisation?
2. Give an advantage of each.
3. Give a disadvantage of each.
4. Name six complications associated with urethral catheterisation.
5. Name two of the exclusion criteria for urethral catheterisation.
6. How often should the following equipment be changed?
    - catheter valve
    - catheter drainage bags
    - catheter 'belly bags'.
7. Is the use of talcum powder and cream recommended?
8. After catheterisation, what information should be recorded in the patient records?
9. Where are CSUs collected from the drainage bags?
10. After a catheter drainage bag has been emptied using an aseptic technique, what should the port be decontaminated with?

KEY POINTS

- Reasons why urinary catheterisation are performed.
- Catheter care.
- Exclusion criteria for urethral catheterisation.
- Drainage bags.
- Problems associated with urinary catheterisation.
- Procedure for male urethral catheterisation.

USEFUL WEB RESOURCES

Cancer Research UK: www.cancerresearchuk.org

Teach Me Surgery. Male urethral catheterisation procedure and aftercare (2018): https://teachmesurgery.com/skills/clinical/male-urethral-catherisation

Geeky Medics. Male catheterisation OSCE guide: https://geekymedics.com/penile-catheterisation-osce-guide
Bard Care UK: https://www.bardcare.uk
NHS - http://www.nhs.uk/conditions/urinary-catheters

REFERENCES

National Patient Safety Agency (2009). *Hospital Alerted to Risks of Inserting Suprapubic Catheters Incorrectly*. London: NPSA.
Rahman, A.A., Lophatananon, A., Brown, S.S. et al. (2010). Hand pattern indicates prostate cancer risk. *Br J Cancer* 104: 175–177.

Chapter 6

FEMALE URETHRAL CATHETERISATION

LEARNING OUTCOMES

By the end of this chapter you will have an understanding of the theory and practice of performing the clinical skill of female urethral catheterisation and have knowledge of the female external catheter device.

WHY IS URINARY CATHETERISATION PERFORMED?

Female urinary catheterisation is performed for the same reasons as male urethral catheterisation – for drainage, investigations and instillations – with the added purpose of:

- emptying the bladder during childbirth.

ANATOMY AND PHYSIOLOGY

Before undertaking the clinical skill of female urethral catheterisation, we need to have knowledge of the female anatomy.

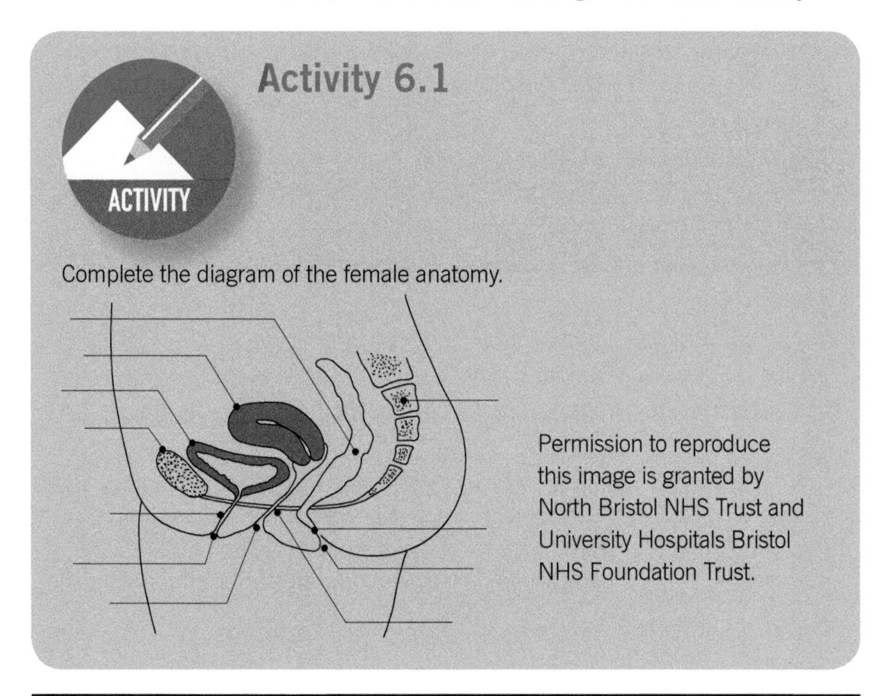

Activity 6.1

Complete the diagram of the female anatomy.

Permission to reproduce this image is granted by North Bristol NHS Trust and University Hospitals Bristol NHS Foundation Trust.

Female catheterisation can be trickier to perform than male catheterisation, as three orifices are quite close together. As a woman gets older, everything appears to move 'south' (i.e. downwards) making finding the urethra, into which we must insert the catheter tube, more difficult to locate, especially if the patient is overweight. It is for this reason that, very often, the catheter tube is inadvertently inserted into the vagina. In this case, as no urine will be flowing out of the catheter, it is best to leave the tube in place until another tube is inserted, hopefully this time into the urethra. Only then do we remove the first tube that went into the vagina.

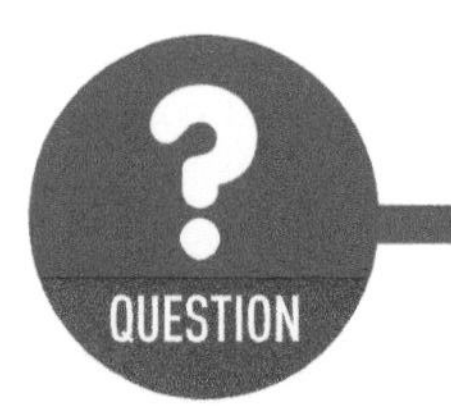

Question 6.1 Why would you leave the catheter tube in place if you know it is not in the urethra?

DID YOU KNOW?

Traditionally, male catheterisation was deemed a higher clinical skill necessitating extended training, while female catherisation was seen as a lesser skill, requiring less training!

Pelvic Floor

The pelvic floor, which males also have, is a set of muscles that stretches like a hammock from the pubic bone in the front to the bottom of the backbone. These firm, supportive muscles help to hold the bladder, womb and bowel in place. The muscles are firm and kept slightly tense to stop urine leakage from the bladder or leakage of faeces from the bowel.

When we pass urine or have a bowel motion, the pelvic floor muscles relax to facilitate this. Afterwards, they tighten again to prevent further movement or leakage.

Over time, the pelvic floor muscles can become weak and sag due to a variety of reasons, such as childbirth, the menopause and hormonal changes, lack of exercise, or obesity, as extra weight puts extra strain on these muscles. As the pelvic floor becomes weaker, urine leakage and/or faecal leakage may then occur, being more evident when women laugh, sneeze or exercise. This can be very embarrassing.

As with any muscle, 'if you don't use it, you'll lose it'.

Pelvic floor exercises can strengthen these muscles and have been found to be particularly effective for stress incontinence (a type of urinary incontinence), improving or even stopping leakage of urine as the muscles become stronger over time.

As health professionals, part of our role is in education, and we may need to inform our patients on techniques to improve the pelvic floor. One technique is shown below.

- This pelvic floor exercise can be done sitting down or standing up. Imagine yourself sitting on the toilet passing urine. Now imagine yourself stopping the flow of urine: really 'pull' upwards and squeeze and stop it. You may find this hard to start with. Some people are able to manage the technique of 'going up' in stages: much like a life going up floors! As you practise this exercise, you can try holding for a few seconds and then relaxing and letting go.
- Now, if you are not already sitting, sit down, with your knees slightly apart. Imagine you are trying to stop yourself passing wind from the bowel. Really squeeze and lift the muscle around your back passage. You should feel the skin around the back passage being pulled up and away from the chair and you should feel the muscle move, but your buttocks and legs should not move.

You can do these exercises at any time, in any place and unless you pulled some strange faces while you were doing them, no one need know! Also, don't worry if you could not feel the muscles very well, as over time the pelvic floor will strengthen and tighten and you will gain more control over them.

Another good exercise to strengthen the pelvic floor, as long as you don't have back, hip or knee pain and discomfort, are pelvic tilts:

- stand with your feet 30cm apart, with your knees slightly bent. Now rotate hips in a clockwise circular movement. Do this for approximately 10minutes every day.

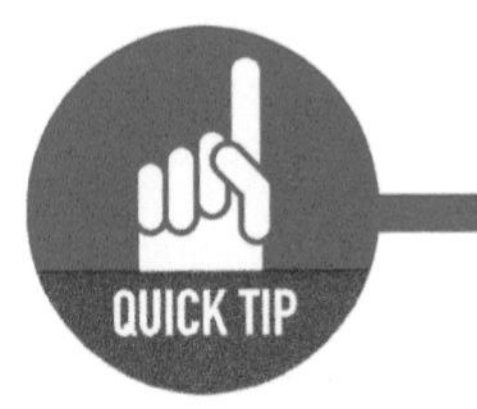

Avoid high-impact-type physical exercises, as these may weaken the pelvic floor muscle. Yoga, pilates, swimming, cycling and belly dancing are considered 'good' exercises to do if you are experiencing bladder weakness.

FLUID BALANCE

Fluid balance is an essential tool in determining hydration.

If there are problems with fluid balance then it may indicate warning signs that the patient is acutely or potentially ill. If fluid balance is not monitored correctly then such signs can be missed, resulting in:

- late referral and missed opportunities
- unexpected deterioration
- prolonged stay in hospital
- in some cases, death.

Note that weighing incontinence pads may not be a problem when recording fluid balance, as this is relatively easy to perform, but weighing sheets may well be difficult. Therefore, practise estimating amounts of any wet sheets on beds using water (empty/unused beds, obviously).

PERSONAL CARE

Good hygiene procedures must be maintained to prevent infection when a patient has a catheter in place. Daily, or more frequent, washing must be undertaken. The gold standard for washing is good, old-fashioned soap and water. The catheter tube should be wiped downwards, away from the body. Sometimes a patient may ask for 'a sprinkling' of talcum powder. This can cause infection as the talc may transgress into the bladder, up along the tubing, and the patient should therefore be dissuaded. However, if a patient has mental capacity, and you have informed them of the rationale for its non-use and they still wish to have some, then you will need to document this fact.

PROCEDURE FOR FEMALE URETHRAL CATHETERISATION

Catheter types are shown in Chapter 5, but it should be noted that shorter, female-length catheters are often no longer used in many clinical areas on men or women, following an alert by the NPSA (National Patient Safety Agency, 2009). Only standard-length catheters are now used in many care settings on both sexes (see Chapter 5 for more details).

Some clinical areas now use catheter boxes whereby all the equipment is contained in a prepacked box. Figure 6.1 shows a catheter box which come in bed-bag, leg-bag and urometer varieties.

The Equipment

- Sterile catheterisation pack.
- Disposable and waterproof pad.
- Sterile and non-sterile gloves.
- Appropriate size and length of catheter.
- Prepacked sterile anaesthetic lubricating gel.
- Appropriate catheter valve and support accessories for catheter bag.
- Light source.
- Sterile water and syringe for the balloon (if not included in catheter pack).

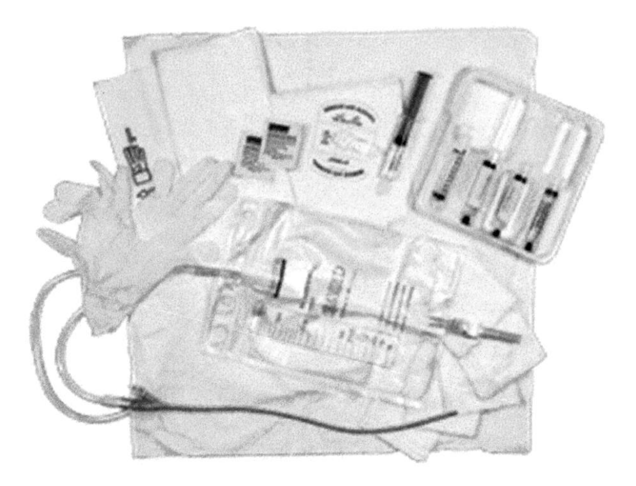

Figure 6.1 Prepacked catheter box.

- Disposable plastic apron.
- Drainage bag and stand or holder if appropriate.
- 0.9% sodium chloride (Normasol sachet).
- Alcohol hand rub.
- Information leaflet/booklet with contact name if appropriate.

Guidelines for Female Catheterisation

1 Explain and discuss the procedure with the patient. Gain consent.

2a Screen the bed. Ensure that you have a good light source. Ask the patient to shower or wash the vulval area with soap and water if able. Otherwise, assist the patient to perform this task.

2b Assist the patient to get into the supine position with the legs extended.

2c Do not expose the patient at this stage of the procedure. Ensure that the patient is warm.

3 Wash hands using soap and water using the six-step hand-washing technique.

4 Clean and prepare the trolley, placing all equipment required on the bottom shelf.

5 Take the trolley to the patient's bedside, disturbing the screens as little as possible.

6. Open the outer cover of the catheterisation pack and slide the pack on to the top shelf of the trolley.
7. Using an aseptic technique, open the supplementary packs. Open catheter into sterile receiver.
8. Remove the cover that is maintaining the patient's privacy and position a disposable pad under the patient's buttocks and thighs.
9. Put on a disposable plastic apron and non-sterile disposable gloves.
10. Assist the patient to get into the supine position with knees bent but apart, hips flexed and feet together.
11. Separate the labia minora so that the urethral meatus is seen. If there is any difficulty in visualising the urethral orifice due to vaginal atrophy and retraction of the urethral orifice, consider repositioning the patient, for example by raising the patient's buttocks, and ensuring that the lighting is good.
12. Clean both the labia and around the urethral orifice with 0.9% sodium chloride (Normasol) using single downward strokes.
13. Remove non-sterile gloves and clean hands using the six-step technique with alcohol gel and put on sterile gloves.
14. Warn the patient of the risk of stinging from anaesthetic gel. First, squeeze a drop of the single-use anaesthetic gel to cover the meatus. Then squeeze the gel into the urethra and discard the tube. Wait for 3–5 minutes.
15. Place the catheter, in the sterile receiver, between the patient's legs.
16. Introduce the tip of the catheter into the urethral orifice in an upward and backward direction. Advance the catheter until urine flows steadily.
17. Check that the catheter is draining properly then gently inflate the balloon according to the manufacturer's instructions.
18. Withdraw the catheter slightly and attach it to a compatible valve or drainage system.
19. Support the catheter by using a specifically designed support strap. Ensure that the catheter does not become taut when the patient is mobilising.

20 Make the patient comfortable. Ensure that the area is dry.

21 If this is the patient's first catheterisation, measure the amount of urine drained after 20 minutes.

Female External Catheter

Medication and surgery aside, up to now, males had the option of urinary sheaths or penile clamps (not used so often today) pad and pants, urinary drainage devices or urinary catheterisation for urinary incontinence. Women had just two choices, pad and pants or urinary catheterisation for urinary incontinence. Is it any wonder that females experienced more moisture lesion problems! Now a new device has been developed, called the PureWick™ Female External Catheter (Bard Medical, Crawley).

The PureWick female external catheter has been designed to address the need for a simple, non-invasive urine management solution for women. The PureWick is a flexible, contoured 'sausage like' device (Figure 6.2) that is positioned between the labia and gluteal muscles, remaining completely external. The PureWick device is then connected to a wall vacuum system (in hospital) or transportable vacuum system (community) operating on low – pressure and continuous suction, which pulls the urine away from the body into a collection cannister and lowers the risk of infection.

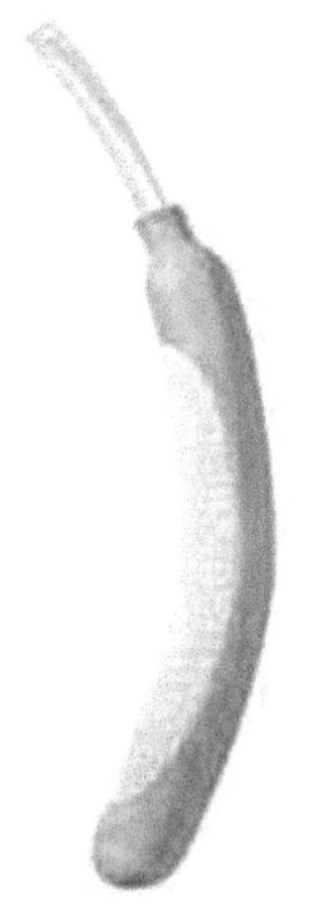

Figure 6.2 The PureWick™ Female External Catheter (Bard Medical, Crawley). Source: Reproduced with kind permission from BD Diagnostics.

The benefits of this system are that it is:

- simple and intuitive – low pressure suction wicks away the urine through the soft material, thus minimising the risk of skin irritation and urine leakage
- non-invasive – reduces the need for indwelling catheterisation and therefore minimises the risk of catheter-associated urinary tract infections
- accurate – provides accurate urine output measurements
- designed for comfort – PureWick is soft, flexible and contoured to function while the user is lying down, seated and/or asleep.

TEST YOUR KNOWLEDGE

1. What is the first thing you must do prior to performing a urethral catheterisation?
2. Where is the pelvic floor sited?
3. What is considered the 'gold standard' when proving catheter care?
4. Why is female urinary catheterisation performed?
5. What is the name of the female external catheter?
6. Is it only females who have a pelvic floor?

KEY POINTS

- The pelvic floor.
- Female anatomy and physiology.
- Fluid balance.
- Procedure for female urethral catheterisation.

USEFUL WEB RESOURCES

Nursing Times. Urinary catheters 2: inserting a catheter into a female patient (2017): https://www.nursingtimes.net/clinical-archive/continence/urinary-catheters-2-inserting-a-catheter-into-a-female-patient-16-01-2017

Teach Me Surgery. Female urethral catheterisation (2017): https://teachmesurgery.com/skills/clinical/urethral-catheterisation-female

Bard Medical. PureWick Female External Catheter: http://www.bardcare.uk/clinicians/view-products/external-catheters/purewick-female-external-catheter

REFERENCE

National Patient Safety Agency (2009). *Hospital Alerted to Risks of Inserting Suprapubic Catheters Incorrectly*. London: NPSA.

Chapter 7

BOWEL CARE

Clinical Skills for Nurses, Second Edition. Claire Boyd.

LEARNING OUTCOMES

By the end of this chapter you will have an understanding of the theory and practice of performing the clinical skill of bowel care management.

Bowel care management includes the assessment and observation of a patient's stools and seeking and/or providing treatment for any dysfunction. Bowel care management may also include the clinical procedures of digital rectal examination (DRE), administration of enemas and/or suppositories, digital removal of faeces (DRF) and digital rectal stimulation (DRS), and risk assessments and contraindications for these procedures, including autonomic dysreflexia (ADR).

Many patients are embarrassed to discuss their bowel function so we are talking about a very sensitive issue. A poor patient with limited mobility is very often expected to 'open their bowels' on a commode, next to their bed, with just a flimsy curtain between them and their neighbour. Mix into the equation the change of diet, change of environment and change of medication (including analgesia, etc.) it is no wonder that some patients get constipated. Worse still is when a patient contracts a healthcare-acquired infection such as *C. diff* (short for *Clostridium difficile*), which causes very smelly diarrhoea!

We first need to look at the basic anatomy and physiology of the bowels and some key basic principles.

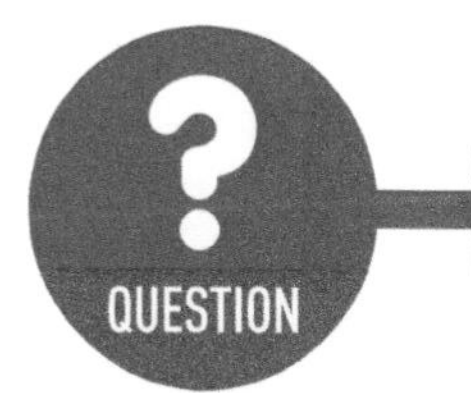

Question 7.1 What do you think are the five main functions of the bowel?

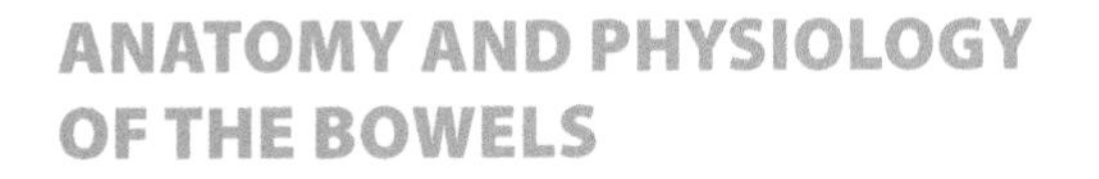

ANATOMY AND PHYSIOLOGY OF THE BOWELS

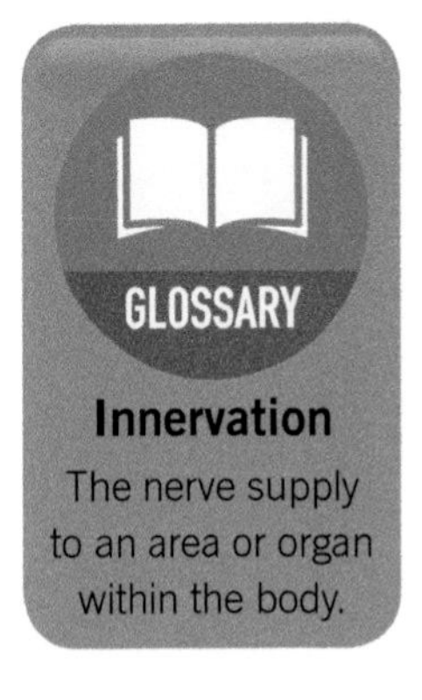

Information from the lower bowel and brain is conveyed via sympathetic (lumbar) and parasympathetic (sacral) nerve roots: the autonomic nervous system. These are the pudendal nerves (from the external genital organs), which carry fibres from the sacral nerves S2–S4 to the pelvic floor muscle and descending colon and rectum.

The sympathetic innervation comes from thoracic nerves T9–T12, and it is these nerves that keep the anal sphincter closed. The parasympathetic nervous system relaxes the anal sphincter when we need to defecate. This voluntary control usual starts at age 18 months, when we learn to control this movement to defecate in the right place and at the right time.

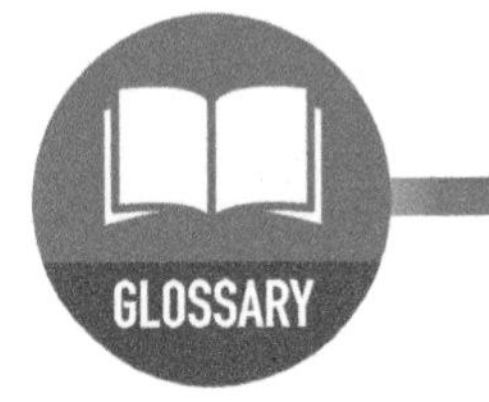

Peristalsis

Wavelike movement along some of the hollow muscular tubes of the body, such as the intestines. Alternate contraction and relaxation of the circular and longitudinal muscle push the contents of the tube forward.

What we eat enters the mouth, thus beginning the digestive process, and travels down the oesophagus and into the stomach (Figure 7.1). From there, the food is broken down by digestive enzymes and the vitamins, proteins, water, etc. are digested and absorbed to be used by the body. The intestinal contents are moved along by peristalsis, taking approximately three to five hours to travel along the small intestine. You may have heard the expression 'gut motility' to describe this movement process.

The matter then travels up the ascending large colon, along the transverse large colon and down the descending large colon, into the rectum to the anal canal and out the anus.

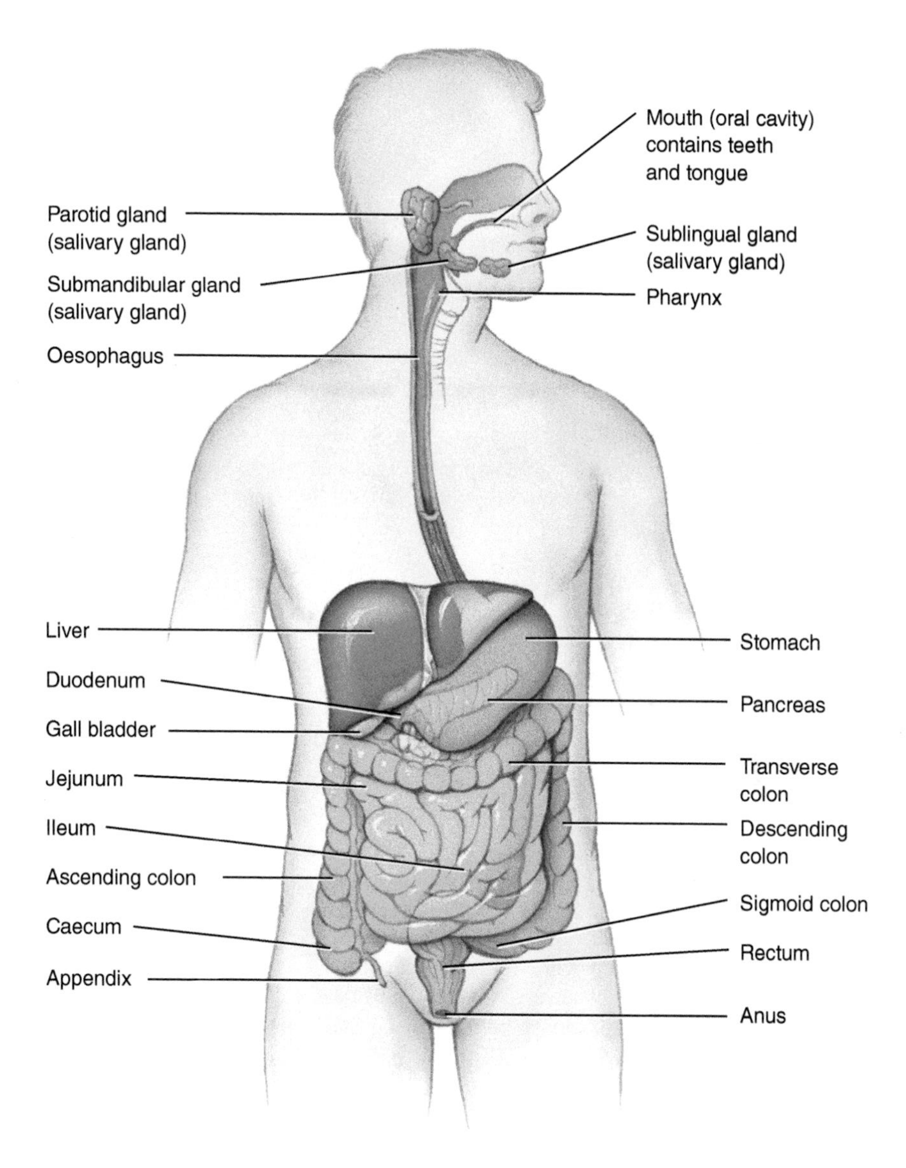

Figure 7.1 The digestive system. Source: Reproduced from Peate and Nair (2020) with permission.

Box 7.1 Definitions of Constipation and Diarrhoea

Constipation may be defined when two or more of the following are present:

- straining or pain when trying to open your bowels
- passing large, dry, hard, lumpy stools
- a sensation of incomplete evacuation of stools
- not having a bowel movement at least three times in the last week
- stomach ache, feeling bloated or sick.

Chronic constipation may be defined as infrequent bowel movements or difficult passage of stools that persists for two weeks or longer.
Diarrhoea may be defined as: the frequent evacuation or the passage of abnormally soft or liquid faeces.

If the faeces are not expelled for some time, they will become hard and more difficult to pass, resulting in constipation. Box 7.1 gives the diagnostic criteria for constipation.

Diarrhoea may be *acute* (usually lasting less than two weeks) and may be caused by an infection, or *chronic* (lasting more than two weeks) and may be due to inflammatory bowel disease. Box 7.1 gives the definition of diarrhoea.

Any bowel dysfunction may have a profound effect on an individual – both physiologically and/or psychologically, and will require a sensitive approach to treat.

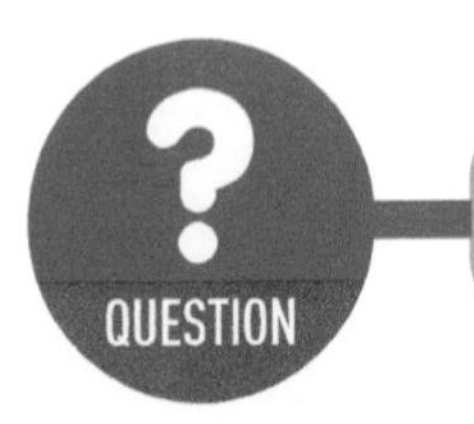

Question 7.2 What do you think are the causes of bowel dysfunction? List five causes.

ASSESSMENT

When assessing any bowel dysfunction, we need to establish the patient's normal bowel pattern, as they may normally produce 'loose' stools, so this is 'normal' for them. Any dysfunction to the normal pattern will then need to be investigated. For a good assessment, we need to look at:

- history of onset (is it linked to any lifestyle or emotional changes? Has the patient recently travelled abroad?)
- normal bowel pattern
- present bowel pattern (also look at consistency and colour of stool and any blood present)
- stool chart recordings (using the Bristol Stool Chart)
- diet and fluid intake (any changes? is the patient adequately hydrated?)
- medication (any changes?)
- understanding/mental capabilities (has the patient become confused?)
- skin breakdown (any changes to perianal or peristomal integrity?)
- mobility (any changes?)
- physical assessment.

THE BRISTOL STOOL CHART

The Bristol Stool Chart was developed by Dr Ken Heaton at the University of Bristol and can be used to evaluate the effectiveness of treatments for various diseases of the bowel. It is also used as an assessment tool to monitor our patients' bowels before any problems occur (Figure 7.2).

Type 1 and Type 2 stools may be difficult to pass due to constipation. We could advise our patients who produce these stools to increase their fibre intake and hydration, if their medical condition allows. This caution is required because increasing dietary fibre (e.g. adding bran to the diet) may lead to faecal loading, slow transit time, increased flatus and increased pain for patients with conditions such as irritable bowel syndrome.

Type 3 and Type 4 stools are considered to be the easiest stool to pass and are therefore the 'ideal' stool.

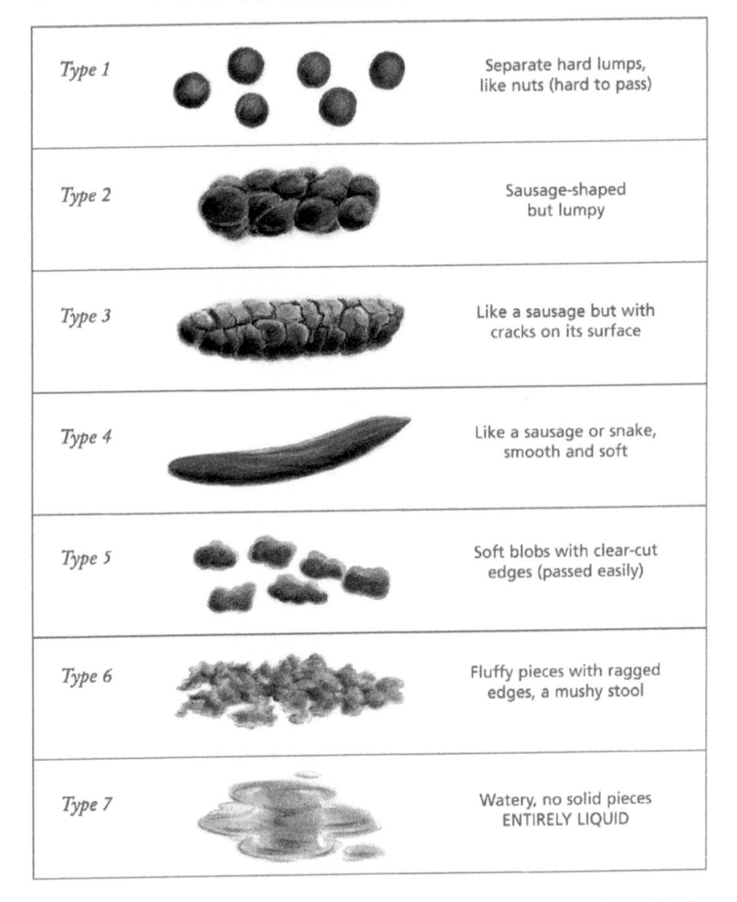

Figure 7.2 The Bristol Stool Chart. Source: Permission to reproduce this image is granted by North Bristol NHS Trust and University Hospitals Bristol NHS Foundation Trust.

Type 5, 6, and 7 stools are tending towards diarrhoea, with type 7 possibly resulting in dehydration, electrolyte imbalance and malnutrition, as well as abdominal pain/cramping and perianal skin breakdown. Patients with ileostomies and colostomies will also need to change their appliances more frequently, possibly causing peristomal skin breakdown.

This assessment tool, which is now used worldwide, is an important part of the whole patient assessment process as, once we have established a dysfunction, treatment can commence. Table 7.1 shows a few of the medications that may be used in the care of bowel dysfunction.

Table 7.1 Medications used in bowel care.

Medication type	Information
Acute diarrhoea	
Antimotility drugs	**Antimotility drugs may be used in the management of uncomplicated acute diarrhoea in adults, but not in young children.**
Codeine phosphate: oral	**Tolerance and dependence may occur with prolonged use.**
Loperamide hydrochloride: oral	**Used in the treatment of acute diarrhoea in adults and children over 4 years of age.**
Morphine: oral	**Causes sedation; risk of dependence.**
Constipation	
Laxatives	**Laxatives may be used in patients with constipation, after it has been established that the constipation is not secondary to an underlying undiagnosed condition. They may be prescribed as an enema or to be taken in oral form.**
Bulk forming	**Bulk-forming laxatives relieve constipation by increasing faecal mass, stimulating peristalsis: ispaghula husk (Fybogel®, Ispagel® Orange).**
Stimulant laxatives	**Stimulant laxatives increase intestinal motility. Excessive use can cause diarrhoea: bisacodyl is an oral medication or presented in suppository format; docusate sodium, oral; glycerol, suppository; senna, oral.**
Faecal softeners	**Enemas containing arachis oil (ground nut/peanut oil) lubricate and soften impacted faeces to promote a bowel action: arachis oil, enema.**
Osmotic laxatives	**Osmotic laxatives increase the amount of water in the large bowel, either by drawing fluid from the body into the bowel or by retaining the fluid they were administered with: lactulose, oral; macrogols (Movicol®), oral.**

A **suppository** is a preparation that may be inserted into a body cavity, such as the rectum or the anus, to be absorbed to treat conditions such as constipation.

A **pessary** is the same, but goes into the vagina to treat conditions such as candidiasis (thrush). As well as a medication, a pessary may also be an instrument or ring to treat conditions such as a prolapsed womb.

An **enema** is fluid that is infused through a tube into the anus to remove faeces or to insert drugs into the rectum.

Many healthcare environments insist that staff administering medications via suppository or as an enema must have received bowel care training and must be assessed as competent to perform this clinical skill.

MEDICATION REVIEW

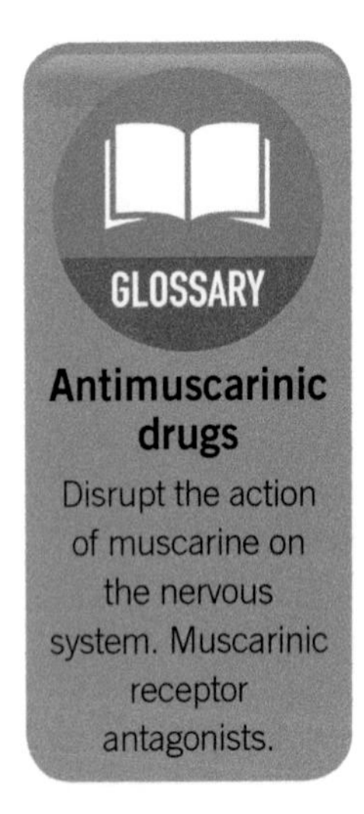

Antimuscarinic drugs

Disrupt the action of muscarine on the nervous system. Muscarinic receptor antagonists.

As part of the patient assessment process, and following an episode of constipation, faecal impaction or faecal incontinence, the patient's medications should be reviewed. This is because many drugs have adverse effects that affect gut motility and stool consistency. The main groups are:

- broad-spectrum antibiotics
- opioids
- antidepressants
- antimuscarinics
- antihistamines
- laxatives
- antidiarrheals
- iron preparations
- obesity medication
- antacids.

CONSTIPATION

We have talked about constipation, but what exactly is it? Well, it most commonly occurs when waste or stools move too slowly through the digestive tract or cannot be eliminated effectively from the rectum, resulting the in the hard lumpy stools we read about in Box 7.1. The main causes of constipation are:

- Not eating enough fibre, such as fruit, vegetables and cereals.
- Not drinking enough fluids.
- Not moving about enough and spending long periods sitting or lying-in bed.
- Being less active and not exercising.
- Often ignoring the urge to go to the toilet.
- Changing your diet or daily routine.
- An adverse effect of medicine.
- Stress, anxiety or depression.

Constipation is also common during pregnancy and for six weeks after giving birth. It may also be more common in the older adult or those with learning disabilities. If you are caring for someone with dementia, or young children, constipation again may be easily missed. It is therefore important to be aware of any changes in those you are caring for in their behaviour that might mean that they are in pain or discomfort. Complications of constipation include:

- **Swollen veins in your anus (haemorrhoids)** – straining to have a bowel movement may cause swelling in the veins around the anus.
- **Torn skin in your anus (anal fissure)** – straining to have a bowel movement can cause tiny tears in the anus.
- **Stools that cannot be expelled (faecal impaction)** – being unable to pass stools may cause an accumulation of hardened stools that become stuck in your intestine.
- **Intestine that protrudes from the anus (rectal prolapse)** – Straining to have a bowel movement can cause a small amount of the rectum to stretch and protrude from the anus.

CHRONIC CONSTIPATION

Complications of long-term constipation can lead to faecal impaction. This is when the stools build up in the last part of the large intestine (rectum). The main symptom of faecal impaction is diarrhoea after a long bout of constipation. Chronic constipation has many possible causes, including not addressing constipation in the first instance. Causes also include:

- Blockages in the colon or rectum which may slow or stop the stool movement.
  Causes: tiny tears in the skin around the anus (anal fissure), colon cancer, narrowing of the colon (bowel stricture), other abdominal cancer that presses on the colon, rectal cancer, rectum bulge through the back wall of the vagina (rectocele).
- Neurological problems can affect the nerves that cause muscles in the colon and rectum to contract and move stool through the intestines.
  Causes: damage to the nerves that control bodily functions (autonomic neuropathy), multiple sclerosis, Parkinson's disease, spinal cord injury, stroke.
- Difficulty with the muscles involved in elimination (e.g. pelvic muscles).
  Causes: the inability to relax the pelvic muscles to allow for a bowel movement (anismus), pelvic muscles that do not coordinate relaxation and contraction correctly (dyssynergia), weakened pelvic muscles.
- Conditions that affect hormones in the body.
  Causes: diabetes, overactive parathyroid glands (hyperparathyroidism), pregnancy, underactive thyroid (hypothyroidism).

HIRSCHSPRUNG'S DISEASE

Those working in the paediatric sector may come across the rare condition known as Hirschsprung's disease. This condition mainly affects babies and young children and occurs when the stools become stuck in the bowels. In this condition, the nerves are missing from a section at the end of the bowel, which means that stools can build up and cause a blockage, which in turn leads to constipation and occasionally a serious bowel infection called enterocolitis.

Hirschsprung's disease is usually picked up soon after birth, but may be as long as one to two years later. Treatment is by surgery. Signs of this condition are as follows.

- In the newborn:
  - failure to pass meconium within the first 48 hours of birth
  - swollen abdomen
  - vomiting green bile.
- In older infants and children:
  - swollen abdomen and tummy ache
  - persistent constipation that does not get better with the usual treatments
  - not feeling well or not gaining much weight.

FIBRE

As we can see, one of the treatments we may advise our patients for the relief of common constipation is to increase their fibre intake. However, a patient once informed me that they have no idea how much fibre they had ingested after eating a lunch of salad. Yes, it can be complicated; many residential and nursing homes have laminated sheets giving this information to their residents/service users and for the healthcare staff. Table 7.2 shows this fibre information table.

Table 7.2 Food fibre amounts.

Food	Serving size	Fibre (grams per serving)
Fruit		
Apple with skin	1 medium	3.7
Apple without skin	1 medium	2.4
Apple sauce	½ cup	2.0
Apricots	3 medium	2.5
Bananas	1 medium	2.7
Blueberries	1 cup	4.0
Cantaloupe melon	1 cup (pieces)	1.3
Cherries	10 cherries	1.3
Grapefruit	½ medium	1.3
Grapes	1 cup	1.2
Honeydew melon	1 cup (pieces)	1.0

(Continued)

Table 7.2 (*Continued*)

Food	Serving size	Fibre (grams per serving)
Orange	1 medium	3.0
Peach	1 medium	1.7
Pear	1 medium	4.0
Pineapple	1 cup (pieces)	2.0
Plum	1 medium	1.0
Raisins (seedless)	⅔ cup	4.0
Raspberries	1 cup	8.4
Strawberries	1 cup	3.4
Tangerine	1 medium	2.0
Watermelon	1 cup (pieces)	0.8
Vegetables		
Baked beans	1 cup	14.0
Broccoli (boiled)	½ cup	2.3
Carrot	1 medium	2.0
Cauliflower	½ cup	1.7
Coleslaw	½ cup	1.0
Corn on the cob	1 ear	2.0
Cucumber	½ cup (pieces)	0.5
Green beans (boiled)	½ cup	2.0
Lettuce	½ cup (pieces)	0.5
Mushrooms	½ cup (pieces)	0.4
Onions (boiled)	½ cup	1.0
Peas, green	½ cup	4.0
Potato (baked with skin)	1 medium	5.0
Potato (boiled)	1 medium	2.0
Potato salad	½ cup	1.6
Spinach (boiled)	½ cup	2.2
Sweet potato (baked)	1 medium	3.0
Tomato, raw	1 medium	1.0

Table 7.2 (*Continued*)

Food	Serving size	Fibre (grams per serving)
Cereals		
All-Bran	½ cup	10.0
Cheerios	1 cup	3.0
Honeynut Cheerios	1 cup	2.0
Multigrain Cheerios	1 cup	3.0
Instant oats	1 pack	3.0
Shredded Wheat	3 biscuits	7.3
Weetabix	10g	3.8
Bread		
Multigrain	1 slice	1.5
White	1 slice	1.0
Wholewheat	1 slice	2.0
Pasta		
Spaghetti	1 cup	6.3
Rice		
Brown rice (long grain)	1 cup	3.5
White rice	1 cup	1.0

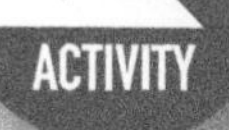

Activity 7.1

Blessing Monye has been feeling 'poorly today' and only managed a light lunch. How many grams of fibre has she ingested?
Single serving of:
Lettuce, cucumber, tomato, coleslaw, baked potato, potato salad and a slice of white bread.

Table 7.3 Fibre amounts required per day.

Age (years)	Fibre amount (g/day)
2–5	c. 15
8–11	c. 20
11–16	c. 25
Adults (>16)	c. 30

Not only is it important to have fibre in our diets to prevent constipation but fibre (often referred to as 'roughage') is also associated with lowering cholesterol levels, heart disease, stroke, type 2 diabetes and bowel cancer.

On average, most adults are only eating 18g of fibre per day, and children and teenagers about 15g or less per day. Table 7.3 shows the fibre amounts we should be ingesting.

BOWEL CARE MANAGEMENT

Once all the initial assessments/treatments have taken place, further investigations may be deemed appropriate. These include:

- DRE
- inserting enemas and/or suppositories
- DRF
- DRS.

These clinical skills are usually job specific (some healthcare assistants may be permitted, after training, to perform a DRE and insert enemas and suppositories) and area specific (in some clinical areas only registered nurses, nursing associates or assistant practitioners, operating department practitioners and medics can perform them). One of these areas is neuroscience, which includes neuro-surgical and neuromedical wards, as these skills are very specialised in this category of patients, (for reasons that we look at in the Autonomic Dysreflexia section of this chapter).

As with all clinical skills, healthcare workers who are able to perform these clinical skills are expected to abide by their local policies and should be conversant with the following standards and guidelines:

- *Bowel Care: Management of lower bowel dysfunction including digital rectal examination and digital removal of faeces* (Royal College of Nursing, 2019).
- *Faecal Incontinence in Adults: Management* (National Institute for Health and Care Excellence, 2007).
- *Guidelines for Management of Neurogenic Bowel Dysfunction in individuals with central neurological conditions.* (Multidisciplinary Association of Spinal Cord Injured Professionals, 2012).
- Management of neurogenic bowel dysfunction in adults after spinal cord injury: clinical practice guideline for health care providers (Johns et al., 2021).

EXCLUSIONS AND CONTRAINDICATIONS

There are certain exclusions and contraindications for performing bowel care management:

- where there is a lack of valid consent from a patient with capacity
- the patient's medical team have given specific instructions that these procedures are not to take place
- the patient has recently undergone rectal/anal surgery or trauma
- rectal bleeding of unknown cause
- malignancy of the perianal area
- ADR.

Specialised care is required in these cases.

RISK ASSESSMENT

The carer should be confident and competent to perform any of these bowel management procedures and a full consultation between the patient and carer should be undertaken to clarify why the procedure is required. A full risk assessment should be performed, looking at specific issues, including:

- *health and safety*: latex, peanuts, etc. allergies
- *documentation*: keep accurate documentation
- *codes of conduct*: patient's dignity, high standards of care, etc.
- *vicarious liability*: always follow employer's guidelines and procedures
- *competence*: are you competent to perform this skill?
- *consent*: cognitive ability, sufficient information, without coercion
- *chaperone*: patient may wish to have a same-sex carer performing this activity (chaperone policies should be adhered to)
- *special precautions and contraindications*: read patient's notes prior to undertaking the procedure and consult with medical staff and/or healthcare colleagues.

Circumstances When Extra Care is Required

It is important to gain all the information you can before undertaking these clinical skills. It is especially important to know the patient's medical history, so you are aware of circumstances when extra care is required, such as:

- active inflammation of the bowel, for example Crohn's disease
- recent radiotherapy to the pelvic area
- rectal/anal pain
- obvious rectal bleeding
- tissue fragility
- if the patient has a history of abuse
- if the patient has a history of allergies
- the patient gains sexual satisfaction from the procedure.

Observations

When performing any of these bowel care management clinical procedures, it is considered best practice to observe vital signs before, during and after the procedure. This is especially important in the neurological patient and for others who may be considered at risk.

DIGITAL RECTAL EXAMINATION

DRE is performed to:

- assess the presence of stool in the rectum, its amount and consistency
- assess the need for rectal medication
- evaluate the efficacy of interventions/medication
- assess anal tone and contraction and its degree.

ADMINISTRATION OF ENEMAS AND/OR SUPPOSITORIES

Indications for the insertion of suppositories or enemas include:

- treatment of inflammatory bowel conditions
- neurogenic bowel dysfunction, as part of a regular bowel management programme
- evacuation of faecal matter from the bowel
- spinal cord injuries, as part of a regular bowel management programme
- drug administration as an alternative to the oral route, to be absorbed for systemic effect.

A DRE should be carried out to assess for faecal loading and for abnormalities including blood, pain and obstruction.

There has been much discussion about whether the blunt end of a suppository should be inserted first so that it is retained for longer. Research by Abd-el-Maeboud et al. (1991) found that this method activates fewer nerve endings in the rectum, allowing it to be retained for longer, otherwise the bodily instincts tell us to push it out as it is a foreign object.

DIGITAL REMOVAL OF FAECES IN ADULTS

DRF may be carried out where other bowel-emptying techniques have failed or are inappropriate, or when the patient has:

- faecal loading/impaction
- incomplete defaecation
- an inability to defaecate
- neurogenic bowel dysfunction, as part of a regular bowel management programme
- spinal cord injuries, as part of a regular bowel management programme.

When performing this clinical skill, it is important not to stretch the anus, so care should be taken to 'hook' the finger when performing this procedure. In spinal patients, a too-rigorous DRF can cause spinal shock.

DRF may be used as an acute intervention following DRE where other methods have failed or as part of the patient's regular bowel management programme. DRF is defined as 'the insertion of a finger into the patient's rectum to evacuate the contents'. It should be avoided if at all possible since it is often distressing to the patient. Cultural and religious beliefs should be considered prior to performing this procedure (Royal College of Nursing, 2019).

DIGITAL RECTAL STIMULATION

DRS may be carried out when the patient has:

- neurogenic bowel dysfunction, as part of a regular bowel management programme
- spinal cord injuries with reflex bowel dysfunction, as part of a regular bowel management programme.

DRS is performed by rotating the finger in the rectum for 15–20 seconds or until the internal sphincter relaxes.

It should not be carried out for more than one minute at a time. This cycle can be repeated up to three times and an anaesthetic gel may be prescribed to ease the process.

AUTONOMIC DYSREFLEXIA

ADR is a syndrome unique to patients with spinal cord injury at the level of the sixth thoracic vertebra or above. It is a sudden, potentially lethal rise in blood pressure and is often triggered by acute pain or harmful stimulus below the level of the injury. It should always be treated as a medical emergency; if left untreated, it can be fatal due to the risk of cerebral haemorrhage, seizure or cardiac arrest.

ADR only affects spinally injured patients. This is why the procedures discussed here can only be performed by experienced registered practitioners (registered nurses) in most clinical areas.

The condition arises as a result of an autonomic (sympathetic) reflex in response to pain or discomfort (noxious stimuli) perceived below the level of the lesion. The reflex creates a massive vasoconstriction below the level of the lesion causing a pathological rise in blood pressure that can be life-threatening if allowed to continue unchecked.

Advanced bowel care for this category of patients can only be performed by staff with specialised knowledge and skill.

Common Causes of Autonomic Dysreflexia

There are many triggers for this condition, such as:

- distended bladder (e.g. catheter blockage or bladder outlet obstruction)
- distended bowel (e.g. constipation, impaction or full rectum)
- ingrown toenail
- fracture below level of the lesion
- pressure ulcer
- contact burn, scald or sunburn
- urinary tract infections or bladder spasms

- renal or bladder calculi
- pain or trauma
- deep vein thrombosis
- overstimulation during sexual activity
- severe anxiety.

Signs and Symptoms of Autonomic Dysreflexia

- Pounding, usually frontal, headache.
- Severe hypertension (spinal cord-injured patients have a lower resting blood pressure).
- Slow pulse.

One or more of the following:

- Flushed appearance of the skin above the level of the injury.
- Profuse sweating above the level of the injury.
- Pallor above the level of the injury.
- Nasal congestion.

Treatment of Autonomic Dysreflexia

Under normal circumstances, a person with tetraplegia may have a low blood pressure (e.g. 60/90 mmHg). A rise to 'normal' levels (80/120 mmHg) may represent a significant elevation. Regular monitoring of blood pressure is essential, as changes can occur quickly; monitor blood pressure every five minutes until blood pressure control is achieved.

ADR is considered a medical emergency and nurses need to ensure that the patient has medication prescribed, such as an antihypertensive (e.g. nifedipine), should this condition occur. Administer the prescribed medication and monitor the patient's blood pressure: if there is no response then call the crash team. Box 7.2 shows the treatment of ADR in more detail.

Note: ADR can usually be easily remedied by the removal of the cause of the painful stimuli, use of local anaesthesia and/or a vasodilator.

Box 7.2 Manifestations, Causes and Treatment for Autonomic Dysreflexia

Manifestations:

- Severe hypertension
- Bradycardia
- 'Pounding' headache
- Flushed or 'blotchy' skin above the level of lesion
- Pallor below the level of lesion
- Profuse sweating above the level of lesion
- Shortness of breath

Common causes:

- Any painful or noxious stimuli below the level of injury
- Distended bladder (usually due to catheter blockage or another form of bladder outlet obstruction)
- Distended bowel (usually due to a full rectum, constipation or impaction)
- Skin problems/ingrowing toenail
- Fracture below the level of lesion
- Labour/childbirth
- Ejaculation (Glickman and Kamm, 1996; Wiesel and Bell, 2004)

Actions to take:

- Sit the patient up (where possible) to induce an element of postural hypotension.
- Ensure that there is adequate urinary drainage (change the catheter if necessary, do not give a bladder washout/instillation).
- Empty the rectum by DRF (local anaesthetic gel should be used).
- Blood pressure should be treated until the cause is found and eliminated (administer a proprietary vasodilator, e.g. nifedipine, as prescribed).
- If unable to locate cause, or symptoms persist, get help immediately.

THE PROCEDURES: STEP BY STEP

Procedural Steps for Digital Rectal Examination

Consider the circumstances when extra care is required, and also the exclusions and contraindications. Before undertaking DRE, abnormalities of the perineal and perianal area should be observed, looking for rectal prolapse, haemorrhoids, anal skin tags, wounds, dressings, discharge, anal lesions, gaping anus, skin condition, bleeding, faecal matter, infestation and foreign bodies.

Equipment required
Disposable latex-free gloves
Incontinence sheet/pad
Wipes
Lubricant (e.g. KY® Jelly)
Waste bag
Plastic apron

Intervention	Rationale
1 Check with patient and hospital notes for any contraindications.	**To minimise risk of potential problems.**
2 Explain the procedure and obtain verbal consent.	**To reduce anxiety and gain consent.**
3 Ensure that the procedure is carried out in the privacy of a cubicle or curtained area.[a]	**To maintain patient's privacy and dignity.**
4 Wash hands with soap and water and put on apron and double gloves.	**To prevent potential contact with body fluids and minimise the risk of cross-infection.**
5 Position the patient on their left side with their back next to the edge of the bed and their knees flexed. Place an absorbent pad under the patient and cover the patient with a sheet.	**Positioning allows ease of entry into the rectum following the natural curve of the colon.**

(***Continued***)

6 Examine the perianal area for any abnormalities before proceeding.	To ensure that it is safe to proceed.
7 Reassure the patient throughout the procedure.	To avoid unnecessary stress or embarrassment and ensure continued consent.
8 Lubricate a gloved index finger and insert gently into the rectum. Note: nurses' nails must be kept short.	To minimise patient discomfort and avoid anal mucosal trauma.
9 Assess for the presence of faecal matter using the Bristol Stool Chart (Figure 4.2).	To check for the presence of faecal matter and to establish the consistency of the stool.
10 Slowly withdraw finger from patient's rectum when finished. Check for presence of faeces or blood on glove.	To minimise patient discomfort.
11 Remove top glove and dispose of in clinical waste bag.	To minimise risk of cross-infection.
12 Wipe residual lubricating gel from anal area.	To ensure the patient's comfort and avoid anal excoriation.
13 Dispose of gloves, apron and equipment into a yellow bag and wash hands.	To prevent cross-infection.
14 Ensure that the patient is comfortable and observe for any adverse reactions.	To and minimise embarrassment and note adverse reactions.
15 Record findings in nursing documentation and communicate findings with medical team if appropriate; consistency, volume, date and time should all be recorded appropriately.	To ensure correct care and continuity of care.

[a] Where available and appropriate, DRE should be performed in the patient's side room to protect the privacy and dignity of the patient and to protect other patients from potential malodour.

Procedural Steps for Administration of Enemas and Suppositories

Consider the circumstances when extra care is required and also the exclusions and contraindications. Before inserting enemas or suppositories, abnormalities of the perineal and perianal area should be observed, as for DRE.

Special precautions also need to be assessed: recent colorectal surgery, malignancy (or other pathology) of the perianal region and low platelet count.

Equipment required
Disposable latex-free gloves
Incontinence sheet/pad
Wipes
Lubricant (e.g. KY Jelly)
Waste bag
Plastic apron
Suppository or enema, prescribed by medic or nurse prescriber

Intervention	Rationale
1 Obtain verbal consent and document it.	To reduce anxiety and gain consent.
2 Collect and prepare the equipment.	To ensure that the procedure is conducted in an efficient and timely manner, thus reducing anxiety.
3 Take patient's pulse rate at rest prior to and during the procedure.	To record baseline pulse and monitor for changes.
4 Take blood pressure in spinally injured patients prior to, during and at the end of the procedure.	To record baseline pulse and monitor for changes.
5 Prepare the patient; assist with removing clothing from waist down, help in positioning patient on left lateral position, knees flexed, taking into consideration the normal line of the sigmoid colon.	Positioning allows ease of entry into the rectum following the natural curve of the colon.
6 Protect bedding and mattress and wash hands with soap and water.	To maintain infection control procedures and patient dignity.
7 Observe the anal area and put on gloves and apron.	To ensure that it is safe to proceed; to prevent potential contact with body fluids and minimise the risk of cross-infection.
8 Lubricate the gloved index finger; inform the patient that you are about to perform the procedure.	To minimise patient discomfort and avoid anal mucosal trauma.

(*Continued*)

9	Gain patient cooperation by asking the patient to relax prior to insertion of index or middle finger.	To avoid unnecessary stress or embarrassment and ensure continued consent.
10	Insert the gloved finger into the anus slowly and on into the rectum.	To minimise patient discomfort and avoid anal mucosal trauma.
11	Assess for faecal matter, document the amount and consistency, using the Bristol Stool Chart (Figure 4.2). Assess the need for medication.	To establish rectal loading and the consistency of the stool.
12	Lubricate the blunt end of the suppository or the tube tip of the enema (after the cap has been removed); inform the patient that you are about to perform the procedure, then insert the suppository/enema via the anus into the rectum.	Inserting the suppository blunt end first allows the anal sphincter to assist with insertion (Abd-El-Maeboud et al., 1991).
13	Clean the anal area; remove gel by wiping residual from area to ensure that it does not cause irritation or soreness.	To maintain cleanliness; to leave patient comfortable.
14	Dispose of equipment as per local policy.	To prevent cross-infection.
15	Help the patient to get up and dressed and into a comfortable position; offer toileting facilities as appropriate.	To maintain dignity and to minimise embarrassment.
16	Document procedure fully on completion.	To establish effectiveness of procedure; to ensure continuity of care.

Procedural Steps for Digital Removal of Faeces

Consider the circumstances when extra care is required and also the exclusions and contraindications. Before undertaking DRF, abnormalities of the perineal and perianal area should be observed, as for DRE. When undertaking this procedure, the following observations and risk factors should be considered and documented, and medical assistance/advice should be sought:

- pulse at rest prior to procedure to obtain a baseline reading
- pulse during procedure
- blood pressure in spinal injury patients prior to, during and at the end of the procedure
- signs and symptoms of ADR (headache, flushing, sweating, hypertension)
- distress, pain, discomfort
- bleeding
- patient collapse.

Equipment required
Disposable latex-free gloves
Incontinence sheet/pad
Plastic apron
Wipes
Lubricant (e.g. KY Jelly)
Soap and water
Clinical waste bag
Stethoscope
Sphygmomanometer
Bedpan/other suitable receptacle for waste

Note: This is a two-person procedure to ensure accurate and timely monitoring of observations during the procedure. Whereas a blood pressure monitor maybe useful in monitoring situations, in this instance manual pulse and blood pressure should be recorded to note rate, rhythm and amplitude.

Intervention	Rationale
1 Check with patient and hospital notes for any contraindications.	**To minimise risk of potential problems.**
2 Explain the procedure and obtain verbal consent.	**To reduce anxiety and gain consent.**
3 Ensure procedure is carried out in the privacy of a cubicle or curtained area.[a]	**To maintain patient's privacy and dignity.**
4 Take the patient's pulse rate at rest prior to the procedure.	**To record baseline pulse and monitor for changes.**
5 Take the baseline blood pressure in all spinal injury patients.	**To record baseline blood pressure and monitor for any changes.**

(*Continued*)

	Action	Rationale
6	Wash hands with soap and water and put on apron and double gloves.	Prevent potential contact with body fluids and minimise the risk of cross-infection.
7	Position the patient on their left side with their back next to the edge of the bed and their knees flexed. Place an absorbent pad under the patient and cover the patient with a sheet.	Positioning allows ease of entry into the rectum following the natural curve of the colon.
8	Examine the perianal area for any abnormalities before proceeding.	To ensure that it is safe to proceed.
9	For patients receiving this treatment on a regular basis, use lubricating gel on the gloved index finger.	To minimise patient discomfort and avoid anal mucosal trauma.
10	As an acute procedure, a local anaesthetic gel may be applied topically to the anal area. Wait for five minutes before proceeding.	To make the patient as comfortable and pain free as possible and to ensure that the anaesthetic gel has time to have the required effect.
11	Do not apply if anal mucosa is damaged. Check for contraindications.	
12	Reassure the patient throughout the procedure.	To avoid unnecessary stress or embarrassment and ensure continued consent.
13	Insert lubricated gloved index finger into the rectum.	To minimise patient discomfort and avoid anal mucosal trauma.
14	Assess for the presence of faecal matter using the Bristol Stool Chart (Figure 4.2).	To establish rectal loading and the consistency of the stool.
15	In type 1 stool (Figure 4.2) remove a lump at a time until the rectum is empty.	To minimise discomfort and facilitate easier removal of stool.
16	In type 2 stool (Figure 4.2), push finger into the middle of the faecal mass and split it. Remove small sections of faeces at a time into appropriate receptacle.	To minimise discomfort and facilitate easier removal of stool.
17	Do not overstretch sphincter by using a hooked finger to remove large pieces of stool.	To avoid trauma to the rectal mucosa and sphincter.

(*Continued*)

18	If top glove becomes very soiled, remove and replace with a new top glove.	To avoid excessive soiling of patient's skin; to maintain cleanliness.
19	Lubricate gloved finger with each change of top glove. Use extra lubrication as required.	To facilitate easier insertion and minimise friction and discomfort.
20	If faecal mass is too hard, larger than 4 cm across, or you are unable to break it up, stop and refer to medical team.	To minimise risk of ADR.
21	If patient becomes distressed, check the pulse again and check against the baseline reading; stop if pulse rate has dropped, patient is distressed or if there is pain or bleeding in anal area. Check blood pressure for patients with spinal injury.	To monitor condition of patient and stop if necessary.
22	When rectum is empty, remove top glove and clean and dry patient's perianal area.	To maintain cleanliness; to leave patient comfortable.
23	Ensure skin is clean and dry. Observe skin on completion of procedure.	To monitor skin condition.
24	Dispose of gloves, apron and equipment into a yellow bag and wash hands.	To prevent cross-infection.
25	Ensure patient is comfortable and check pulse (and blood pressure for patients with spinal cord injury).	To observe for any adverse reactions.
26	Record bowel results in nursing documentation and communicate results with patient/career and medical team if appropriate. Consistency, volume, date and time should all be recorded appropriately. Report any abnormal findings immediately.	To establish effectiveness of procedure; to ensure continuity of care.

[a] Where available and appropriate, DRF should be performed in the patient's side room or assisted bathroom to protect the privacy and dignity of the patient, and protect other patients from potential malodour.

Procedural Steps for Digital Rectal Stimulation

Consider the circumstances when extra care is required, and also the exclusions and contraindications. Before undertaking DRS, abnormalities of the perineal and perianal area should be observed, as for DRE. The following observations and risk factors should be considered and documented, and medical advice sought:

- pulse and blood pressure should be recorded before, during and after the procedure
- signs and symptoms of ADR in spinally injured patients
- distress, pain, discomfort
- patient collapse.

Equipment required
Disposable latex-free gloves
Incontinence sheet/pad
Plastic apron
Wipes
Lubricant (e.g. KY Jelly)
Soap and water
Waste bag

Intervention	Rationale
1 Check with patient and hospital notes for any contraindications.	**To minimise risk of potential problems.**
2 Explain the procedure and obtain verbal consent.	**To reduce anxiety and gain consent.**
3 Ensure procedure is carried out in the privacy of a cubicle or curtained area.[a]	**To maintain patient's privacy and dignity.**
4 Wash hands with soap and water and put on apron and double gloves.	**Prevent potential contact with body fluids and minimise the risk of cross-infection.**
5 Position the patient on their left side with their back next to the edge of the bed and their knees flexed. Place an absorbent pad under the patient and cover the patient with a sheet.	**Positioning allows ease of entry into the rectum following the natural curve of the colon.**

(***Continued***)

6 Examine the perianal area for any abnormalities before proceeding.	To ensure that it is safe to proceed.
7 Reassure the patient throughout the procedure.	To avoid unnecessary stress or embarrassment and ensure continued consent.
8 Lubricate gloved index finger and insert to the second joint of finger only.	To minimise patient discomfort and avoid anal mucosal trauma.
9 Gently rotate the finger in a clockwise motion for 15–20 seconds or until the internal sphincter relaxes. Note that circular motion originates from the wrist, not the finger.	To trigger reflex relaxation of internal sphincter and promote emptying of the rectum; the pad of the finger to the first joint stimulates reflex relaxation.
10 Do not stimulate for more than one minute.	To prevent damage to anal sphincter.
11 Stop if severe spasms of the anal sphincter occur or if patient shows signs of ADR.	Patient safety.
12 Remove finger to allow faeces to pass.	To allow evacuation to take place.
13 Stimulation cycle can be repeated up to three times.	To facilitate complete evacuation.
14 Check the rectum for the presence of faeces. Proceed to manual evacuation if faeces are present but no faeces have been passed.	To ensure complete evacuation.
15 Remove top glove and clean patient's perianal area with soap and water.	Reduces risk of cross-infection and ensures patient comfort.
16 Ensure that the anal area is clean and dry. Observe skin on completion of procedure.	To prevent infection, contamination and excoriation of perianal area.
17 Dispose of gloves, apron and equipment into a yellow bag and wash hands with soap and water.	To prevent cross-infection.

(*Continued*)

18 Ensure that the patient is comfortable and observe for any adverse reactions.	**To and minimise embarrassment and note adverse reactions.**
19 Record bowel results in nursing documentation and communicate results with patient/carer and medical team if appropriate. Consistency, volume, date and time should all be recorded appropriately.	**To establish effectiveness of procedure; to ensure continuity of care.**

[a]Where available and appropriate, DRS should be performed in the patient's side room or assisted bathroom to protect the privacy and dignity of the patient, and protect other patients from potential malodour.

TEST YOUR KNOWLEDGE

1. Name two functions of the bowel.
2. What is the stool assessment chart called?
3. What is DRE?
4. What does ADR stand for?
5. Name four trigger factors for ADR.
6. What is the purpose of digital rectal stimulation?
7. What are four complications of constipation?
8. How many grams of fibre should a child aged two to five years ingest?
9. How many grams of fibre should an adult ingest?
10. Is stress a main cause of constipation?

KEY POINTS

- Anatomy and physiology of the digestive system.
- The Bristol Stool Chart.
- Medications used in bowel dysfunction.
- Constipation
- Risk assessment.
- Performing a DRE.
- DRF.
- DRS.
- Causes and treatment of ADR.

USEFUL WEB RESOURCES

Royal College of Nursing. Bladder and bowel care: www.rcn.org.uk/clinical-topics/bladder-and-bowel-care

NHS England. Hirschsprung's disease: https://www.nhs.uk/conditions/hirschsprungs-disease

NHS England. Constipation: https://www.nhs.uk/conditions/constipation

Bladder & Bowel UK: www.bbuk.org.uk

REFERENCES

Abd-El-Maeboud, K.H., el-Naggar, T., el-Hawi, E.M. et al. (1991). Rectal suppository common sense and mode of insertion. *Lancet* 338: 798–800.

Glickman S & Kamm MA (1996). Bowel dysfunction in spinal-cord injury patients. *Lancet* June 15:347 (9016):1651–3.

Johns, J., Krogh, K., Rodriguez, G.M. et al. (2021, 2021). Management of neurogenic bowel dysfunction in adults after spinal cord injury: clinical practice guideline for health care providers. *Top Spinal Cord Inj Rehabil* 27: 75–151.

Multidisciplinary Association of Spinal Cord Injured Professionals (2012). *Guidelines for Management of Neurogenic Bowel Dysfunction in Individuals with Central Neurological Conditions.* Humlebaek, Denmark: Coloplast A/S.

National Institute for Health and Care Excellence (2007). Nice: Faecal Incontinence in Adults: Management https://www.nice.org.uk/guidance/CG49.

Peate, I. and Nair, M. (2020). *Fundamentals of Anatomy and Physiology: For Nursing and Healthcare Students*, 3e. Chichester: Wiley.

Royal College of Nursing (2019). *Bowel Care: Management of lower bowel dysfunction including digital rectal examination and digital removal of faeces. Guidance for Nurses.* London: Royal College of Nursing.

Wiesal P & Bell S (2004). Bowel dysfunction: Assessment and Management in the Neurological Patient. In Norton C, Chelvanayagam S (eds) Bowel Continence Nursing, Beaconsfield p181–203.

Chapter 8

STOMA CARE

LEARNING OUTCOMES

By the end of this chapter you will have an understanding of the theory and practice of providing nursing care to individuals with colostomies, ileostomies and urostomies.

Before we look at digestive and renal stomas, we first need to revisit the basic normal anatomy and physiology of these systems.

GLOSSARY

Caecum
The first part of the large intestine. The appendix is attached to the caecum.

THE DIGESTIVE SYSTEM

The human digestive system, simplified, is a complex series of organs and glands that process the food that we eat by breaking them down into smaller molecules. The digestive process begins in the mouth by the action of salivary enzymes breaking down carbohydrates in our food. The food that we eat forms a bolus that, when swallowed, travels along the oesophagus into the stomach by a series of wave-like motions (called peristalsis). Once in the stomach, the food is churned around, partly digested and bathed in gastric acid to produce chime.

Food then enters the duodenum, the first part of the small intestine, travels to the jejunum and then the ileum (the final part of the small intestine). All the while, pancreatic enzymes, bile (from the gall bladder) and enzymes produced by the inner wall of the small intestine continue the process of food breakdown (Figure 8.1).

Food then passes into the large intestine through the caecum, where water and electrolytes are removed from the food. Digestive bacteria such as *Bacteroides, Lactobacillus acidophilus, Escherichia coli* and *Klebsiella* assist in the digestive process. Food travels up into the ascending colon, along the transverse colon and down the descending colon into the sigmoid colon (part of the large intestine between the descending colon and the rectum). Solid waste is then stored in the rectum until it is excreted from the anus.

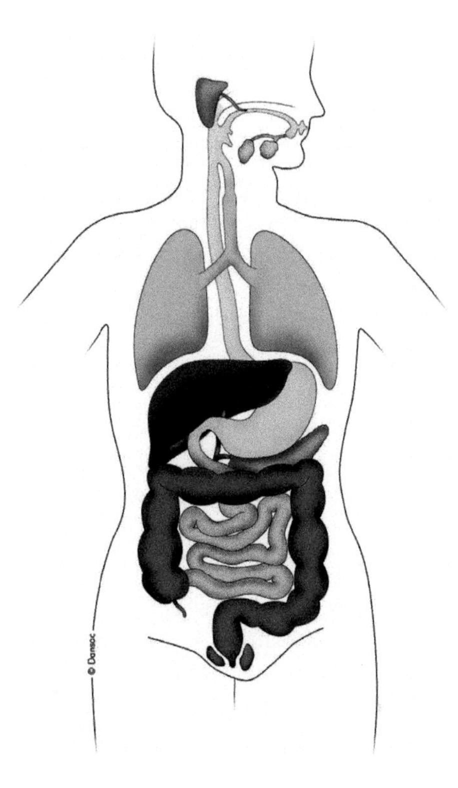

Figure 8.1 The human digestive system. Source: Permission to use this image has kindly been given by Dansac Limited.

THE RENAL SYSTEM

Urine is made in the kidneys and is propelled into the bladder via two tubes, called ureters. Urine is then stored in the bladder, which passively expands to receive the urine. The bladder is composed of interlaced smooth muscle, known as the detrusor muscle. Two sphincters control the bladder outlet: the internal sphincter (controlled by the autonomic nervous system) and the external sphincter (under voluntary control). As the bladder expands and pressure on the sphincters increases, the ureters are compressed, stopping any backflow of urine. Stretch receptors in the detrusor muscle signal that we need to void

Micturition
The process by which urine is expelled from the bladder.

(pass urine) and the internal sphincter opens. The external sphincter then relaxes and micturition occurs.

WHAT IS A STOMA?

A *stoma* is a generic term for 'orifice' or 'mouth' in Greek. An artificial opening or passageway for faeces to be expelled from the small intestine (also known as the small bowel), through the muscle and out through the skin, is known as an **ileostomy**. A similar artificial opening or passageway from the large intestine (also known as the large bowel) is known as a **colostomy**.

The surgery consists of bringing part of the bowel (either large intestine or small intestine) to the surface of the abdomen to form the stoma.

Faeces have now been diverted and will not be expelled through the rectum and anus but out through the stomal opening (although small amounts of mucus may still be expelled here). As the faeces travel along the intestine they change; the matter should generally become more formed as it passes through the bowel. Faeces from an ileostomy are more liquid and have a stronger odour due to the presence of the enzymes involved with food breakdown. In a colostomy, the faeces are more formed, being more solid, as they have undergone more of the digestive process.

A stoma in the renal system is called a urinary diversion; also known as a **urostomy**. This is because urine is diverted away from the bladder. Other types of renal stoma are the **ileal conduit** and **nephrostomy**.

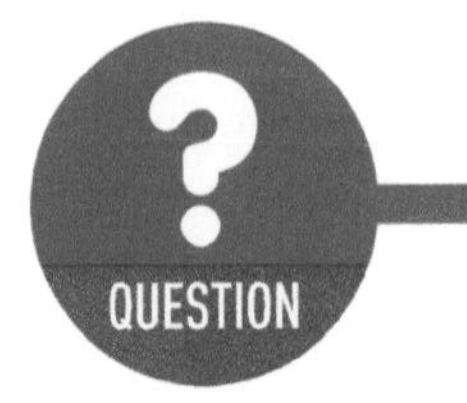

Question 8.1 What is an ileal conduit and what is a nephrostomy?

After surgery for a colostomy, ileostomy or urostomy the sphincter muscles are bypassed. There is no control over bowel movement and a collection device must be worn.

STOMA APPEARANCE

The stoma itself should be warm, moist and red to dark pink in colour (like cheek mucosa). Patients sometimes call the stoma a 'bud' or 'strawberry' because of its colour and shape. This bud is very vascular, meaning that it will bleed profusely if cut. However, the patient will not feel this as the intestine has no nerve endings. The skin around this bud is known as the peristomal skin and will feel pain if the skin becomes damaged in any way.

Regardless of the type of surgery – bowel or renal – patients are referred to a specialised stoma care nurse who will advise and support the patient.

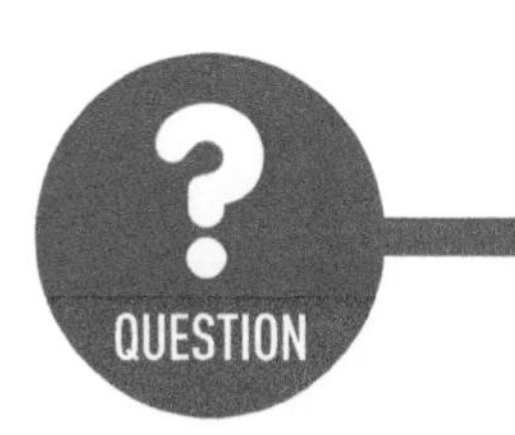

Question 8.2
Fill in the missing words:
Bowel stomas:
Large bowel diversion =
Small bowel diversion =
Renal stomas:
Urinary diversion =

REASONS FOR STOMA SURGERY

For a variety of reasons, stoma surgery may be permanent or 'reversible'. It may be carried out for many medical conditions, including:

- irritable bowel syndrome (bowel)
- ulcerated colitis (bowel)
- cancer (bowel or urinary)
- diverticulitis or Crohn's disease (bowel)
- trauma (bowel or urinary)
- neurological damage (urinary or bowel)
- cancer of the pelvis (urinary or bowel)
- congenital disorder (urinary or bowel).

A reversible procedure is where the two cut ends are reattached, with any damaged or diseased area cut out. Not all patients are able to undergo a reversal operation.

DRAINAGE DEVICES

As the bodily waste (faecal matter or urine) now travels out of the body via the stoma, a collection device will need to be placed at the end of the stoma and attached to the body. Figure 8.2 shows an ileostomy drainage device attached to the skin.

Pouches, Flanges and Wafers

There are various types of collection device. There are two main types of pouch:

- **single use:** used when the skin is in good condition (Figure 8.3)
- **drainable:** changed every four to five days or sooner if outside of bag becomes soiled (Figure 8.4).

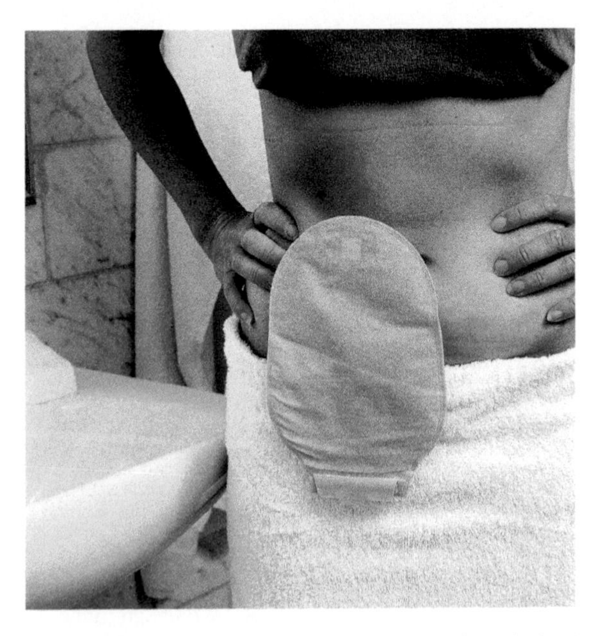

Figure 8.2 Ileostomy stoma device. Source: Permission to use this image has kindly been given by Dansac Limited.

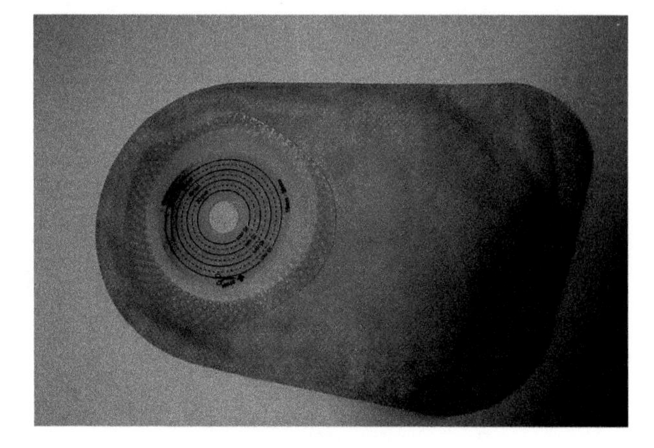

Figure 8.3 A single-use drainage bag.

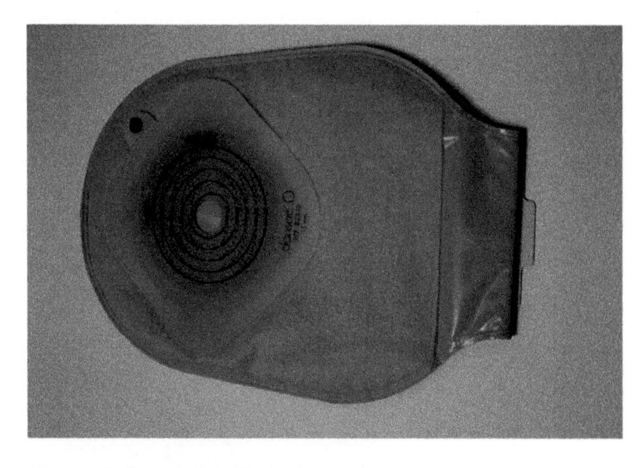

Figure 8.4 A drainable drainage bag.

Urostomy drainage systems have taps at the bottom of the bag, much like urinary catheter drainage bags, to empty the contents.

Pouches can be applied directly to the skin or used with a device known as a flange, on to which the bag can be attached and detached as required. The flange can remain in place for four to five days (Figure 8.5).

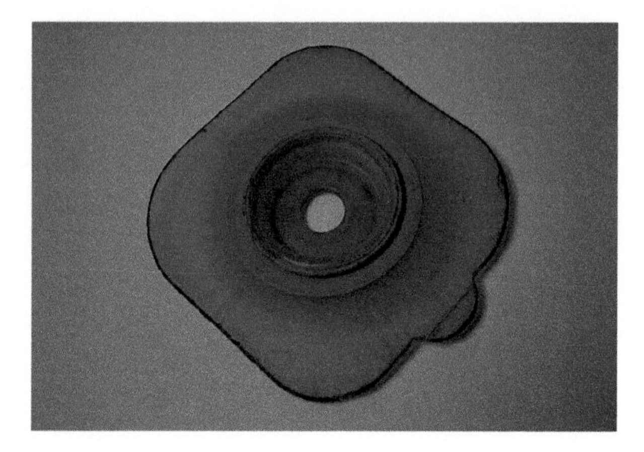

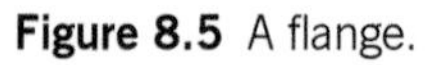

Figure 8.5 A flange.

Pouches may have Velcro or clips to keep the contents in the bag, which can be undone or removed to empty the contents. Digestive stomas may also be covered with a device known as a 'wafer' or 'plaster', which may be used if the individual wishes to go swimming or partake in sexual intercourse. Afterwards the wafer can be removed and a drainage device then reapplied (Figure 8.6).

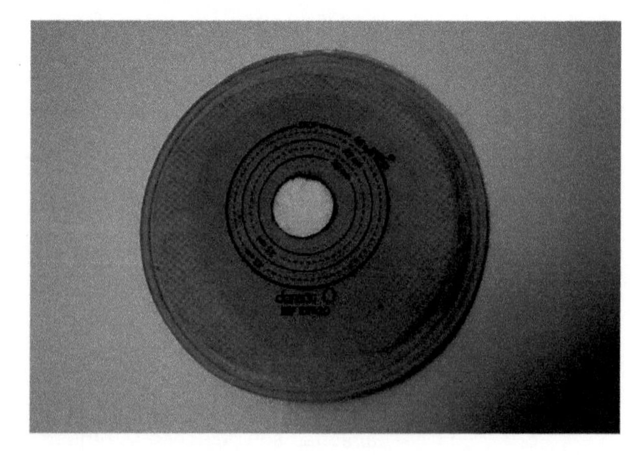

Figure 8.6 A wafer.

Stomas can be budded, flat, oval or round, and stoma drainage systems can be convex or concave depending on the bud (whether an 'innie' or an 'outie'). When preparing a new bag for attachment, the stoma is measured with a measuring gauge and the hole on the bag is cut to size after softening any sharp edges. For example, if the measuring gauge shows that the stoma is 30 mm, then the bag gets cut to this size on the bag. The bag has different sizes printed on it to show where to cut for a particular size. A stoma can change in size as a result of weight gain or loss. The pouch should be warmed in the hands first to enable better bag adhesion and pliability. Patients who have had their stomas for many years tend not to change the stoma size to a great degree so they patients may well receive precut bags by prescription.

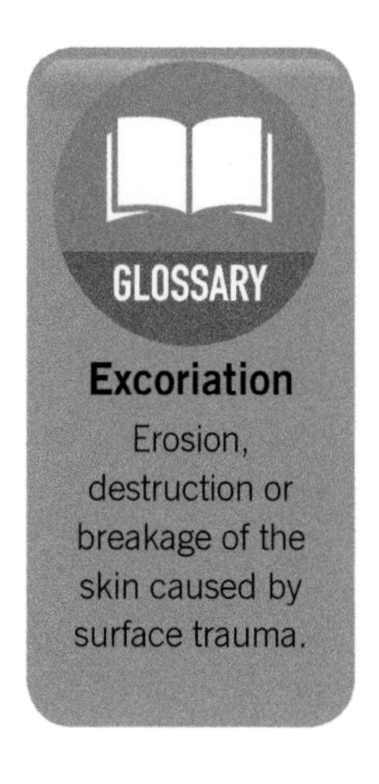

Excoriation
Erosion, destruction or breakage of the skin caused by surface trauma.

SKIN CONDITION

The peristomal skin should be healthy. If it becomes red, sore or excoriated, you must report it immediately to the nurse in charge or district nurse as appropriate. Only specialised products can be applied to the peristomal skin, as products like Sudocrem® do not allow the drainage bag to stick to the skin. The registered nurse overseeing your practice may wish the patient to be referred to a specialised stoma care nurse.

BODY IMAGE

Clients and patients may be worried about their body image. They may ask you for advice regarding sexual activity and my advice was always 'Go for it'! It is best to empty the drainage device before you start. An accident with a burst drainage bag could have very unpleasant results.

It is always best to encourage the individual to empty their own drainage bags as a means of promoting self-care. However, not all clients have the cognitive function or dexterity to perform this activity. In such cases, the career must never show any revulsion when assisting with stoma or renal drainage, as this can adversely affect a patient's psychological wellbeing.

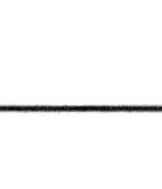

CHANGING A STOMA BAG

Drainage bags should be emptied into a lavatory or a container prior to removal. If they are able, get the patient to sit as far back on the toilet seat as possible and empty the contents down the lavatory. Alternatively, the patient may prefer to stand or kneel, whichever is easiest.

When the bag has been emptied it can be removed, very gently, while holding the skin taut. The peristomal area will need to be cleaned with soap and water and dried well. A new drainage device can be applied after being measured using a measuring gauge and cut to size for a tight fit. Full personal protective equipment (apron and gloves) should be worn if you are carrying out this procedure.

DISPOSAL OF THE STOMA BAG

In a clinical setting, the stoma bag should be disposed of in a clinical waste bag. In the community, the bag should be wrapped in a plastic bag and then wrapped in a second bag. It can then be disposed of in a household waste bin if the client does not have a dedicated waste bin. As already mentioned, the urine and faecal matter should be emptied down the toilet first as you cannot discard human waste with normal household waste.

BIODEGRADABLE DRAINAGE BAGS

New drainage bags on the market have both an inner liner and flange made with biodegradable materials, meaning they are 'flushable'. This material can be flushed in domestic toilets, septic tanks and single-flush siphonic systems. This means that the outer pouch stays clean and can therefore be disposed of in a standard bin, with the stoma output being flushed away in the inner lining.

ISSUES TO CONSIDER

After ileostomy surgery, the patient may experience water and electrolyte loss, so fluids must be well maintained to prevent dehydration. In addition, after any digestive ostomy surgery, digestion and absorption of medicines may be affected. In such cases the patient will require a full review of their medicines.

Urinary tract infections are common in individuals who have undergone urostomy surgery. Preventive measures include drinking plenty of fluids and emptying the pouch regularly.

Certain foods, such as mushrooms, sweetcorn, dried fruit and tomato skins, may cause blockages in an ileostomy. These foods may need to be cut into smaller pieces during preparation.

TEST YOUR KNOWLEDGE

1. Name two types of urinary stoma.
2. What does peristomal skin mean?
3. Give four reasons why someone may require stoma surgery.
4. What should only specialised products be applied to the peristomal skin area?
5. True or false: all stoma drainage devices cannot be flushed down the toilet.
6. True or false: stomas are painful to touch.
7. True or false: an ileostomy is to do with the large intestine.
8. True or false: a colostomy is to do with the small intestine.
9. *Escheric coli* is a type of digestive bacteria.
10. Faeces in the colostomy are more formed than those formed in the ileostomy.

KEY POINTS

- The digestive and renal systems.
- Different types of stoma.
- The appearance of a healthy stoma.
- The rationale for stoma surgery.
- Drainage devices.
- Peristomal skin condition.
- Body image after stoma surgery.
- Changing and disposal of drainage bags.
- Issues to consider after stoma surgery.

USEFUL WEB RESOURCES

Association of coloproctology for Great Britain and Ireland: www.acpgbi.org.uk

CliniMed UK: www.clinimed.co.uk

National Institute for Health and Care Excellence. Stoma care: https://bnf.nice.org.uk/treatment-summary/stoma-care.html

Colostomy UK. Caring for someone with a stoma: https://www.colostomyUK.org/information/information.for.carers

Guts UK: https://gutscharity.org.uk

Bowel Cancer UK: www.bowelcanceruk.org.uk

Dansac UK: www.dansac.co.uk

Chapter 9

TRACHEOSTOMY CARE

LEARNING OUTCOMES

By the end of this chapter you will have an understanding of the theory and practice of performing the clinical skill of tracheostomy care.

A tracheostomy is an opening made in the anterior wall of the trachea to facilitate breathing (Figure 9.1) and may be performed to:

- bypass an upper airway obstruction, such as a tumour, congenital abnormality or trauma, including head and neck or maxillofacial surgery
- assist prolonged ventilation due to a neuromuscular disorder, coma or respiratory failure.

Before we start, you may want to reacquaint yourself with some of the terminology we used in relation to respiration in Chapter 2, such as hypoxia and hypercapnia.

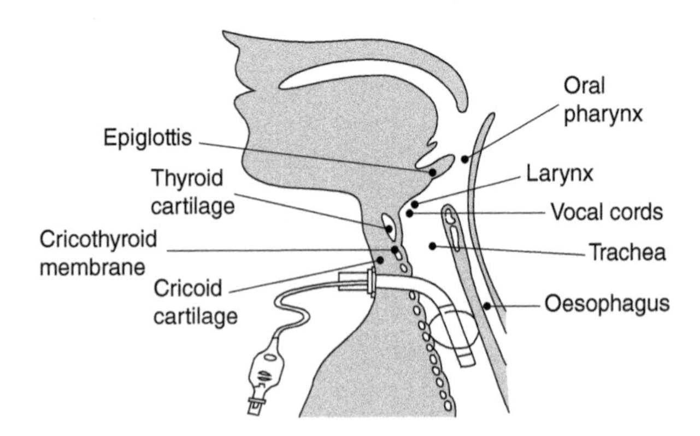

Figure 9.1 Placement of a tracheostomy tube in the trachea. Source: Permission to reproduce this image is granted by North Bristol NHS Trust and University Hospitals Bristol NHS Foundation Trust.

ANATOMY AND PHYSIOLOGY

The effect of bypassing the upper airway (Table 9.1) when a patient has a tracheostomy in place is that the inspired air is not warmed, humidified or filtered. The lower respiratory system is outlined in Table 9.2.

Table 9.1 The upper airway.

Nose	Air is drawn into the nasal cavity and is warmed and humidified so that it reaches the core temperature and saturation in the lungs. The inspired air is also cleaned and filtered to make it free of contaminants.
Pharynx	Three parts: nasopharynx, oropharynx and laryngopharynx.
Epiglottis	This large piece of cartilage moves down and forms a lid over the airway when swallowing, so that food enters the oesophagus and not the larynx. Usually, if anything other than air enters the larynx, the cough reflex is triggered to expel the foreign matter.
Larynx	Contains the vocal cords (which have an avascular, pearly white appearance): air passes over the vocal cords to make the sounds used in speech and other vocalisations.

Table 9.2 The lower respiratory system.

Trachea	Continuation of the larynx: approximately 11.5 cm in length and 2.5 cm in diameter. It starts at the lower border of the cricoid cartilage (the only complete circle of cartilage) and ends at the bifurcating level of the bronchus. The lumen is kept open by incomplete cartilaginous rings. The thyroid gland lies lateral to the trachea. The gland is attached to the trachea by dense connective tissues.
Carina	Where the trachea divides into two main bronchi. Can be damaged by poor suctioning technique.
Right and left bronchus, and bronchioles and alveoli	Alveoli are made up of approximately 300 million cells, which possess thin walls to allow gaseous exchange. Alveoli contain oxygen, but during disease may become porous and filled with blood, bacteria and pus; this may create a crackling sound during inspiration and/or expiration.
The lungs	The right lung consists of three lobes. The left lung consists of two lobes and is a little smaller than the right lung, as it needs to make room for the heart to squeeze in.

The mucociliary transport system is the lining that extends from the nasopharynx to the respiratory bronchioles. This is the only fully functional mechanical barrier against inhaled or aspirated contaminants for patients with tracheostomies. It consists of three layers:

1 Ciliated epithelial cells.
2 Cilia and aqueous layer.
3 Mucus layer.

Contaminants are moved by the cilia as they become trapped in the mucus layer. Cilia have hooked ends and beat with a wavelike movement. This mucus layer must be moist and not too thick, otherwise the contaminants will be too difficult to move; therefore they must have **humidification**. Without humidification, oxygen causes moisture and heat loss, resulting in thick secretions and what we call 'plugging', which may be difficult to clear from the airways.

The optimal temperature of the lungs is 37°C. This equates to a humidity of 44 mg/l (100%).

If the temperature is only 36°C, then the humidity is 42 mg/l. At 35°C, the humidity is 40 mg/l and at 30°C it is 30 mg/l.

If the humidity is anything less than saturated, the cilia are unable to beat and the gel layer loses moisture. If the temperature of the lungs is lower than the core temperature, the cilia beat less frequently and the relative humidity of the inspired air will be lost, resulting in pooling of mucus in the airway. If less than optimal humidification continues, then cell damage occurs and the cilia die. Remember that hospital piped oxygen is colder in the winter, so you may need to raise the temperature slightly.

It is for this reason that humidification must be artificially supplemented to assist normal function and facilitate secretion removal for the patient with a tracheostomy. It is important to assess the adequacy of the selected humidification system at least two hourly. Additionally, it is important to keep the patient systemically hydrated and maintain an adequate fluid intake, which must be increased during periods of infection.

TRACHEOSTOMY TUBES

There are many different types of tracheostomy tube, such as:

- cuffed tracheostomy tube
- uncuffed fenestrated tracheostomy tube
- adjustable-flange tracheostomy tube
- cricothyroidotomy or mini-tracheostomy tube.

Cuffed Tracheostomy Tube

The advantage of the cuffed design (Figure 9.2) is that when the cuff is inflated, it prevents gas from escaping around the tube, enabling assisted ventilation and respiratory support. It also reduces the risk of large-volume aspiration of pharyngeal and gastric secretions into the trachea and lungs, and nosocomial pneumonia. When the pilot balloon is deflated, the cuff is deflated. The cuff pressure is usually measured every six hours.

Note: a speaking valve must never be placed on a cuffed tracheostomy tube. The tracheostomy cuff is made of a soft plastic, which, when inflated, exerts low pressure on the trachea wall.

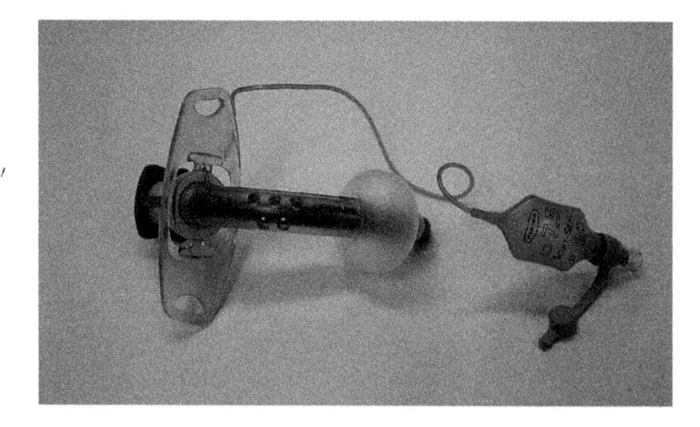

Figure 9.2 A cuffed tracheostomy tube.

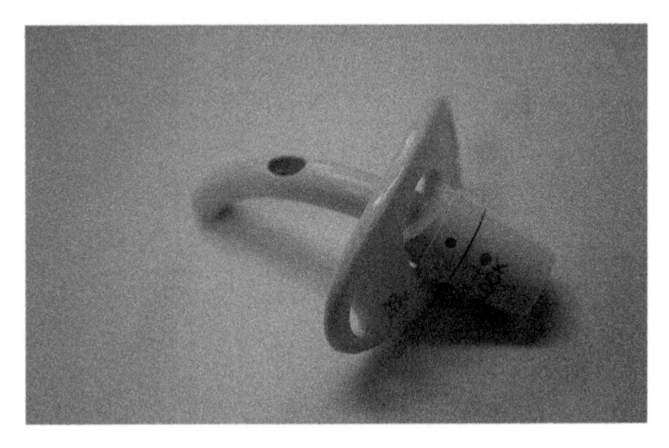

Figure 9.3 An uncuffed tracheostomy tube.

Uncuffed Fenestrated Tracheostomy Tube

The advantage of the uncuffed fenestrated design (Figure 9.3) is that the tube has fenestrations (holes) in the shaft of the tube. These holes direct airflow to pass through the patient's nasal/oral pharynx as well as the tracheostomy during breathing. This facilitates weaning the patient off the tube.

Note: when suctioning is required an inner tube without fenestrations should be inserted prior to the procedure.

Adjustable Flange Tracheostomy Tube

The advantage of the adjustable flange design is that patients with deep-set tracheas (e.g. secondary to obesity, distorted anatomy due to oedema or musculoskeletal deformity such as kyphoscoliosis) can have the tube adjusted to the desired length. These tubes are normally cuffed.

Cricothyroidotomy or Mini-Tracheostomy Tube

The advantage of the cricothyroidotomy or mini-tracheostomy type of tube is that is can be inserted by non-surgeons for life-threatening airway obstruction in emergency situations. It can be used in patients experiencing sputum retention and requiring regular suctioning. Laryngeal function is preserved, including coughing, speaking and swallowing, and natural humidification is not disrupted.

Most tracheostomy tubes are changed every 28 days, or according on the manufacturer's instructions, by experienced surgeons or staff.

Inner Cannula

Tracheostomy tubes may come as a one-piece tube or as a two-piece, meaning that it has a inner cannula. An inner cannula:

- allows maintenance of tube patency
- can be quickly removed if blocked
- facilitates less frequent tracheostomy tube changes due to secretions being cleaned from the inner cannula, thus not building up on the tube itself.

An inner cannula reduces the diameter of the lumen of the tube, which may increase the patient's breathing workload. The inner cannula is usually cleaned every six hours and replaced every seven days.

SUCTIONING TECHNIQUE

Patients require suctioning when they are unable to effectively clear their airway. Suctioning is required to remove secretions with minimal tissue damage and hypoxia (Box 9.1).

Extra consideration as to whether suction is appropriate should be given in the following circumstances:

- pulmonary oedema (use caution: consider the cause)
- hypoxia unless caused by secretions or a blocked tracheostomy tube
- cardiovascular instability
- uncontrolled clotting/international normalised ratio (see Chapter 11)
- severe bronchospasm.

Note: seek guidance from a senior nurse, physiotherapist or doctor.

Box 9.1 Patient Assessment to Indicate Suctioning

Signs/symptoms:

- Abnormal respiratory pattern:
  - Increased respiratory rate
  - Accessory muscle usage
  - Increased work of breathing
- Changes in secretions:
  - Increased quantity: infection,
  - Increased tenacity: inadequate humidification
  - Colour: infection, trauma (blood-stained)
- Persistent coughing
- Change in skin colour:
  - Cyanosis/clammy
- Visible or audible secretions
- Anxiety/agitation

Note: patient assessment should include a full ABCDE assessment (see Chapter 3).

Equipment

Patients with a tracheostomy *must* have the following equipment for performing suction available at their bedside prior to arrival on the ward/unit:

- suction canister
- suction tubing (change at least once a week or when heavily soiled: infection control direction)
- suction catheters of correct size (see below for guidelines)
- Yankauer sucker for oral care (single use only)
- gloves
- aprons
- eye protection
- sterile water (change at least every 24 hours)
- small bowl with lid (change at least every 24 hours)
- oxygen, tubing and tracheostomy mask
- clinical waste bag for disposal of clinical equipment.

Table 9.3 Quick reference to catheter size.

Tube inner diameter (mm)	Suction catheter size (Ch or Fr)
6	8–10
7	10–12
8	12–14
9	14

Suction Catheter Size and Suction Pressure

Choosing a suction catheter of the right size (Table 9.3) is essential for safe and efficient suctioning. The external diameter of the suction catheter should not be greater than half of the internal diameter of the tracheostomy tube.

The pressure of the suction should be at 60–150 mmHg when suction is applied. Greater pressures may cause atelectasis.

If secretions are very tenacious then an increase in the suction catheter size is recommended, rather than increasing the vacuum pressure above 150 mmHg.

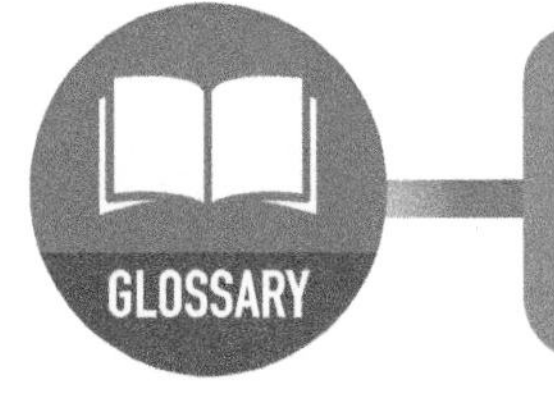

Atelectasis

Failure of part of the lung to expand due to immature cells lining the alveoli (i.e. in premature babies) or damage.

Procedure

1. Inform the patient of the procedure and gain informed consent.
2. Check that the suction is on and working, and set to correct pressure.
3. Wash hands and apply apron and goggles.
4. If the existing cannula is fenestrated, change to a plain inner cannula.

5. Attach the suction catheter to the suction tubing using a clean technique.
6. Place clean gloves on your hands or place a second glove on your dominant hand if gloves are already worn. Do not touch anything other than the unsheathed catheter with the glove on the dominant hand.
7. Remove catheter from sheathing using a clean technique, aiming not to touch the end third of the catheter.
8. Maintain the patient's oxygen in place wherever possible.
9. Gently insert the catheter into the tracheostomy tube without suction applied, until either a cough is stimulated or resistance of the carina is felt.
10. The catheter should be then withdrawn 0.5–1 cm before suction is applied.
11. Withdraw the catheter slowly with suction applied continuously. The catheter should not be rotated.
12. Reapply oxygen if required and observe and reassess patient. Allow the patient to recover before repeating the procedure if required.
13. Inspect the secretions prior to disposing of catheter and gloves and flush through suction tubing with sterile water. (Suction catheters are single-use only.)
14. Change the inner cannula back to fenestrated if required.
15. Evaluate the effectiveness of suctioning and document and report as required.

Note: suctioning should last no longer than 10–15 seconds from insertion to removal of the catheter.

Complications of suctioning can be seen in Table 9.4.

CUFF PRESSURE MONITORING

It is recommended that the cuffs of the tracheostomy tube are maintained at a pressure of 20–25 mmHg (unless instructions state otherwise). Lower pressures prevent optimal ventilation. Higher pressures can compress mucosal capillaries, which can lead to ischaemia and tracheal stenosis. The pressure should be checked every six hours with a designed for purpose pressure gauge.

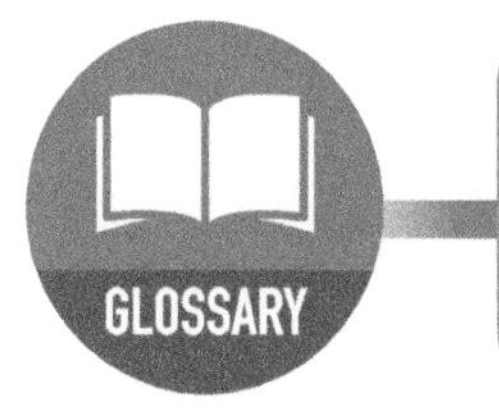

Maceration

Softening of a solid, such as skin softening and damage. Excoriation. Destruction and removal of skin or an organ due to scraping, chemicals or other means.

Table 9.4 Complications of suctioning.

Complication	Potential causes	Action
Hypoxia	Prolonged suctioning and by removing the oxygen given by the tracheostomy mask.	Consider 'staging' suction Episodes. Preoxygenate. Liaise with physiotherapist/medical staff.
Mucosal trauma (e.g. bloodstained secretions)	Poor suction technique.	Consider 'measured-depth' suctioning: use the measurements on a suction catheter to measure the depth of the carina. After this only insert subsequent catheters to 1 cm less than the depth of the carina. Gain expert advice.
Infection	Insertion of a contaminated suction catheter.	Revise technique. Inform medical staff.
Anxiety	Stress and discomfort of being suctioned and enforced coughing.	Reassure and explain necessity.
Pain	Poor technique and 'jabbing the carina' or pain at sites of surgery due to coughing.	Revise technique. Gain medical opinion if pain continues.
Cardiac arrhythmias	Vasovagal response caused by tracheal stimulation by catheter, or severe hypoxia.	Inform medical staff. Consider preoxygenation.
Raised intracranial pressure	Stimulation of trachea causing coughing.	Stagger frequency of suctioning.

(***Continued***)

Table 9.4 (*Continued*)

Complication	Potential causes	Action
Secretions are not clearing easily	Lack of humidification/ patient hydration.	Consider reviewing humidification/ patient hydration, or using saline nebulisers (consult physiotherapist/medical staff).
Patient has pain that is limiting coughing	Pain.	Review analgesia.
Patient has high levels of anxiety related to suction		Inform and reassure.
It is difficult to pass a suction catheter down the tracheostomy tube	Build-up of secretions in inner cannula. If secretions are absent, consider tracheal stenosis or granuloma: request an ear/nose/throat review urgently.	Remove inner cannula for duration of suctioning only.

PROCEDURE FOR CLEANING AND DRESSING THE TRACHEOSTOMY STOMA SITE

The stoma site should be clean and dry to minimise the risk of skin irritation and infection. Secretions collected above the tracheostomy tube cuff may ooze out of the surgical incision and stoma site, leading to skin maceration and excoriation. This increased moisture may act as a medium for bacterial growth and/or prevent the stoma site from healing. This area around the stoma site is called the peristomal.

The stoma site should be assessed at least once every six hours, for trauma, infection or inflammation. Findings should be recorded in the tracheostomy care plan and any problems should be reported as necessary to the senior nurse and/or the doctor.

If Velcro tapes are used, they should be assessed at least every four hours because, when wet, these tapes may stretch, allowing the tracheostomy tube to dislodge. A two-finger technique should be used to secure tube (see procedure, below).

The dressing and tapes may need to be changed more frequently (e.g. if they become soiled).

The cleaning and dressing of the tracheostomy stoma site is a two-person task to prevent dislodgement of the tracheostomy, and if required during an emergency situation.

Red, excoriated or exuding stomas should be swabbed and the doctor informed. Advice should be sought from the wound care team for the treatment of complicated wounds.

Ensure that the patient has had adequate analgesia prior to the procedure, as patients may experience pain and discomfort during the dressing change.

Some tracheostomy tubes are secured with sutures and some may have stay/rescue sutures in place. These sutures require attention upon cleaning, as they are potential sites of infection.

Guidelines for cleaning and dressing the tracheostomy stoma site

Action	Rationale
1 Ensure two people are available prior to undertaking the procedure.	**By removing the tracheostomy tapes, the tracheostomy tube may dislodge. One practitioner therefore holds the tube in place while the other performs the procedure.**
2 Check emergency equipment.	**To ensure patient safety if the tracheostomy tube dislodges.**
3 Explain procedure to the patient and reassure them.	**To ensure that the patient understands the procedure, cooperates and gives consent, and to reduce patient anxiety.**

(***Continued***)

Action	Rationale
4 Check suction equipment.	To ensure patient safety if the patient requires tracheal suctioning during procedure.
5 Screen bed space.	To ensure patient privacy.
6 Wash hands. Put on apron and gloves.	To reduce the risk of cross-infection.
7 Position the patient with their neck slightly extended (if patient's medical condition allows).	To allow easier access to the stoma site and maintain optimum airway alignment.
8 Put on goggles and perform tracheal suctioning, if required.	To reduce the risk of cross-infection from the patient's secretions
9 Wash hands. Don clean apron.	To prevent infection.
10 Prepare dressing trolley using aseptic technique.	To ensure the technique is as clean as possible and all equipment is easily accessible.
11 Unfasten oxygen mask: assist the practitioner to hold it in place over tracheostomy site while at the same time holding the tracheostomy tube in place.	To ensure that patient's oxygen requirements are maintained, to ensure tracheostomy tube is stabilised and to reduce the risk of dislodgement.
12 Remove Velcro tape or ties and old dressing.	To facilitate replacing with new tape/ ties and dressing and to reduce infection.
13 Discard soiled Velcro tape/ties and dressing into clinical waste bag.	To reduce the risk of cross-infection (refer to waste management policy).
14 Assess tracheostomy stoma site for signs of trauma, infection, inflammation and/or maceration. Take a swab if any signs of infection.	To detect and treat stoma complications early to reduce the risk of deterioration of the stoma site.
15 Clean gently around stoma site with 0.9% sodium chloride and gauze. Dry thoroughly.	To remove secretions and crusts; to reduce trauma to tracheostomy site (other cleaning agents may cause irritation to the tracheal mucosa and surrounding skin); to reduce the risk of infection.

Action	Rationale
16 Apply Lyofoam® (Mölnlycke, Vienna) absorbent dressing (or similar) keyhole dressing, starting from below the stoma, placing dressing pink side uppermost.	To ensure the patient's comfort by minimising the risk of pressure, shearing and friction from the tracheostomy tube.
17 Secure in place with ties and tracheostomy foam tube holder or Velcro tracheostomy tape. The tape/ties should be tight enough to keep the tracheostomy tube securely in place but loose enough to allow two fingers to fit between the ties and neck. If using Velcro tape to secure, assess four-hourly.	To promote patient comfort and reduce trauma from a migrating tracheostomy tube; to minimise the risk of reduced cerebral blood flow from the carotid arteries due to excessive external pressure; to assess Velcro tapes are not wet, which may cause stretching to the tapes and tracheostomy tube to become dislodged.
18 Refasten oxygen mask and reposition patient for comfort.	To prevent the risk of hypoxia; to promote patient comfort.
19 Dispose of all soiled equipment.	To prevent the risk of cross-infection.
20 Record procedure and stoma site assessment in patient's notes and/or care plan. Report to doctor and refer to wound care team if further action is required.	To facilitate communication and evaluation: optimal care requires a multiprofessional approach.

TEST YOUR KNOWLEDGE

There may have been some words used in this chapter that you have not come across before and not understood. Did you look these words up in a medical dictionary?

1. What do the following words mean?
   - tenacious
   - bifurcating
   - kyphoscoliosis
   - INR
2. What size suction catheter should normally be used for a 6 mm inner diameter tracheostomy tube?
3. What pressure reading is required for a cuffed tracheostomy tube?

4 When assessing a peristomal site, what does maceration mean?
5 Is persistent coughing an indication for suctioning in a tracheostomy patient?

KEY POINTS

- Anatomy and physiology of the upper and lower airways.
- Tracheostomy tubes.
- Suctioning techniques and complications.
- Cleaning and dressing the tracheostomy stoma site.

USEFUL WEB RESOURCES

National Tracheostomy Safety Project: https://tracheostomy.org.uk

NHS. Tracheostomy: https://www.nhs.uk/conditions/tracheostomy

Great Ormond Street Hospital for Children. Living with a tracheostomy: https://www.gosh.nhs.uk/conditions-and-treatments/procedures-and-treatments/living-tracheostomy

Chapter 10

POINT-OF-CARE TRAINING

LEARNING OUTCOMES

By the end of this chapter you will have an understanding of the theory and practice of performing the clinical skill of point-of-care training: urinalysis, faecal occult blood testing and blood glucose monitoring.

Point-of-care training is when we conduct pathology testing at the 'point of care' – that is, in the clinical area – rather than sending the sample (e.g. blood, urine, faeces) in the first instance to the biochemistry laboratory to be tested. Some areas call this 'near-patient testing'.

Note: all these tests require training and assessment before you are able to perform the procedures.

ACTIVITY

Activity 10.1

Before we get started, let's test your knowledge of urine to see how much you know.

1. What is the pH value of healthy urine?
2. What might a low urine pH value indicate?
3. To what might a low urine pH indicate a predisposition?
4. What might a high urine pH value indicate?
5. What is the most common cause of a high urine pH reading?

URINALYSIS

There are many urine-testing sticks on the market (Figure 10.1); they are sometimes referred to as 'dip sticks' or reagent strips. The ones that we shall be looking at are called Combur® 5 and Combur 7 (Roche), but the technique and

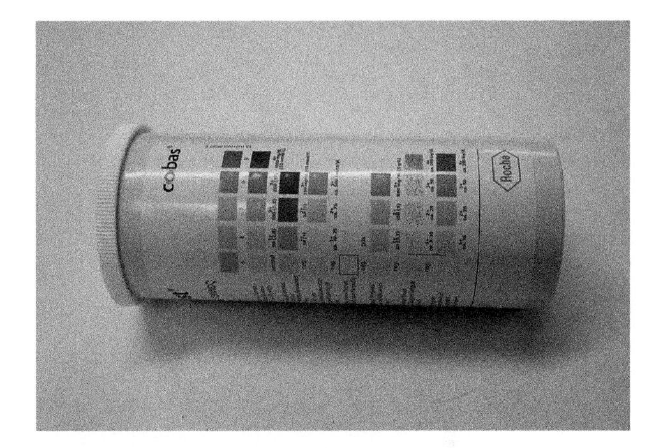

Figure 10.1 Urinalysis test strip container.

overview is predominately the same whichever testing kit you use. You will, of course, need to check the instructions given by the testing kit's manufacturer.

It should be remembered that all patient samples are a potential infection risk and health and safety procedures must be adhered to, including disposal of used materials.

The Combur 5 urine test strip is used to detect urine pH and the presence of glucose, ketones, proteins and blood or haemoglobin in the urine sample. The Combur 7 urine test strip is used to detect the urine pH, plus glucose, ketones, leucocytes, nitrite, protein and blood. Figure 10.1 shows the container for these test strips.

To perform the test, you will require a test strip kit, your fob watch for timing, an apron and gloves, and a paper hand towel or two. You will also require a collection container. There are a few prerequisites to performing this test; one is to check that the test strips have been stored correctly with the cap intact, out of direct sunlight and away from extremes of temperature. The other is that the person conducting this test must not be colour blind.

The Sample

The sample must be collected in an uncontaminated container; this means something that has not been cleaned with disinfectant. Foil or paper mâché containers are ideal for this type of sample collection; the patient's details should be written on the container. The best urine to collect for this test is an early morning urine sample, collected midstream. Your patient may not know what this means, so you may need to explain it to them, as well as asking them to clean the genital area before providing the sample. Children and immobile patients may need assistance with sample collection.

For detection of diabetes, a sample collected roughly two hours after a meal is preferred. A urine sample should not be tested more than two hours after it has been produced, and should not contain blood, faeces, cream, etc., as these will contaminate the sample and the test will have to be repeated. Once a sample has been obtained and mixed well, the assessment begins. First, we inspect the colour and smell.

The Test

1. Wash and dry your hands and put on gloves and apron. Ensure that you have a good light source under which to conduct this test.
2. Check the expiry date of the strips on the container and that the cap still contains loose desiccant (indicating that the test strips are not damp). If the desiccant in the cap is not loose (i.e. it is in one large clump) it may be indicative that dampness has contaminated the test strips.
3. Remove a test strip from the container. Hold the white end of the test strip and inspect the test pads. The pads should look slightly lighter than the left-hand lines of pads on the colour chart on the strip container.
4. Immerse the pads in the urine sample for no longer than one second (Figure 10.2 – step 1).
5. Remove the test strip from the urine by dragging the reverse side of the test strip over the edge of the sample container to remove the excess urine (Figure 10.2 – step 2).
6. Place the test strip face up on a paper towel (Figure 10.2 – step 3; check that the towel does not contain high levels of starch).
7. Wait for exactly 60 seconds.

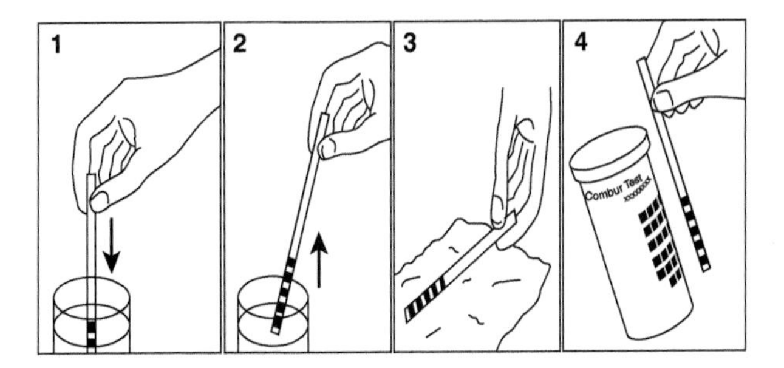

Figure 10.2 Urinalysis procedure. Source: Permission to reproduce this image is granted by North Bristol NHS Trust and University Hospitals Bristol NHS Foundation Trust.

8. Read the test strip against the colour chart on the test strip container immediately after the 60 seconds are up (Figure 10.2 – step 4). The colour will continue to develop: if the time has gone beyond 120 seconds then discard the strip and repeat the test.
9. When reading the strip, make sure that it is orientated correctly and that the pads line up with the correct portions of the colour chart. The pad nearest the holding strip should be in line with the pH chart.
10. Results: for each pad select the colour block on the chart that most closely matches the pad.

Record all the parameters measured: the pH and results and numbers from each of the pads. The results from a test shown in Figure 10.3 would need to be recorded and reported. They show:

- pH 5
- Glucose +3
- Ketones +2
- Leucocytes +1
- Nitrite – negative
- Protein +2
- Blood – negative

If the patient's results are not consistent with their condition, retest with a freshly collected sample. Box 10.1 highlights the issues to consider when checking a urinalysis result.

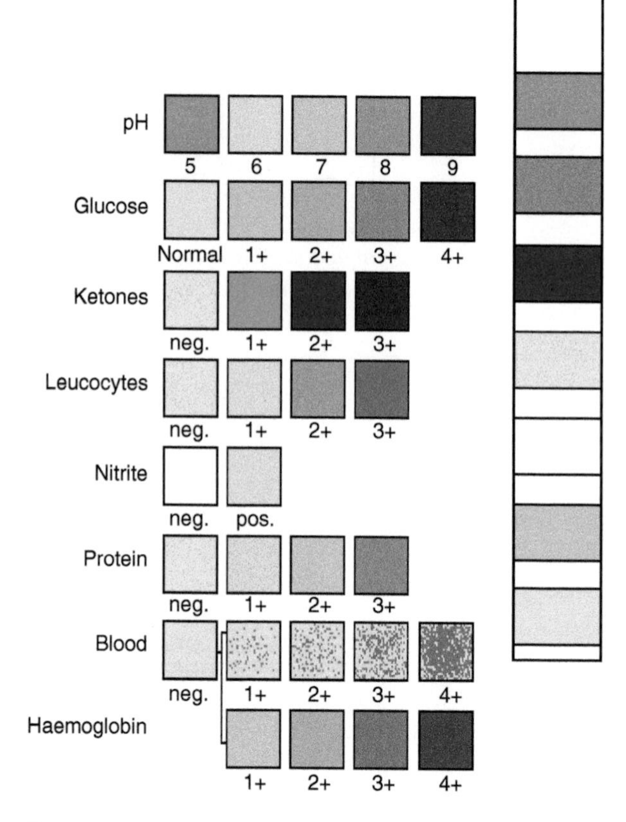

Figure 10.3 Urinalysis results. Source: Permission to reproduce this image is granted by North Bristol NHS Trust and University Hospitals Bristol NHS Foundation Trust.

What does It All Mean?

Depending on the test kit you are using, urinalysis can be used to show early signs and symptoms of many diseases, such as:

- liver disease
- renal disease
- diabetes mellitus

Box 10.1 Issues to Consider when Checking Urinalysis Results

- Diet, medication or disease may alter the colour or smell of the urine. Some drugs, foods or infections can colour the urine, e.g. co-danthramer, beetroot, red blood cells (red), methylene blue (green), rifampicin (red-orange), nitrofurantoin, bilirubin (deep yellow), L-dopa, metronidazole (red brown) and *Pseudomonas* infection (blue-green). Foul-smelling or cloudy urine may indicate infection. Stale-smelling (ammoniacal) urine may be due to stagnation.
- If the patient is not clean, the urine may be contaminated and an incorrect result reported.
- Blood may be present due to menstruation. Allow two days before and two days after menstruation.
- The test strips should only be used on urine samples and not any other type of fluid (pleural fluids, knee fluids, cerebral spinal fluid, etc.).
- The blood/haemoglobin pad colour may be reduced by excess proteins or by an infected urine sample.
- The pH will be falsely elevated if the urine has been left longer than 2 hours before the test is performed.
- The protein may be falsely positive if the pH is below 5 and falsely negative if the pH is above 9.
- Vegetarians often have a pH that is above 9.
- Ketones can be present after a long fast. Ignore any red colour on the pad. High doses of salicylate will reduce the colour.
- If glucose is positive for a person who has *not* been diagnosed with diabetes, further investigation is required.

- hypertension
- pre-eclampsia
- biliary disease
- renal stones
- malignant tumours.

Glucose is not normally present in urine and its presence may indicate that renal absorption is abnormal or that the patient has raised blood glucose levels.

Ketones in the urine may indicate uncontrolled diabetes or anorexia.

Protein in the urine may indicate hypertension, pre-eclampsia, glomerulonephritis, infection or diabetes.

Blood in the urine may indicate infection, renal stones, injury to the renal tract or kidneys or malignancy.

Nitrite may be indicative of infection. The sample of urine for this test should be obtained from urine passed four hours after the last voiding, or should be an early morning sample.

Bilirubin in the urine may indicates hepatic disease.

FAECAL OCCULT BLOOD TEST

As with urine testing, there are many different test kits on the market to test for faecal occult blood. The one we look at here is the Hema-Screen™ (Immunostics) test kit. The test is designed to detect the presence of abnormal amounts of blood in the faeces.

Faecal *occult* blood testing just means that the blood may not be apparent to the naked eye: hence the use of chemical slides to detect the 'hidden' blood.

This test is useful in the assessment of patients with gastrointestinal symptoms with anaemia and is used in screening asymptomatic patients for colorectal cancer.

To perform the test, you will require a test kit (containing the test slides, developer and applicator), your fob watch, apron, gloves, collection container for the sample and some paper towels. Figure 10.4 shows the test slide.

The test kit should have been stored correctly, away from extremes of humidity. Again, as with urine testing the person conducting the test must not be colour blind.

The sample should be fresh and should be collected in a container that has not be cleaned with disinfectant; foil or paper mâché containers are ideal. Whichever type of container is used, it must have the patient's details clearly

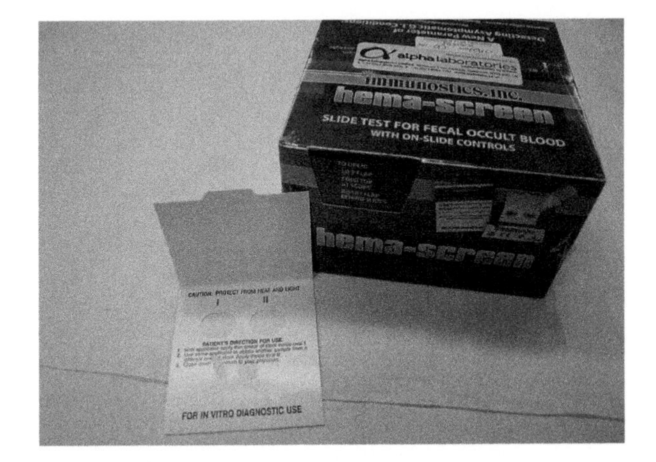

Figure 10.4 Faecal occult blood testing slide.

written on. We need to inform our patient that the sample must be free from urine or any other potential contaminants, with the genitals cleaned prior to sample collection. Some patients may require assistance with the sample collection.

Dietary Preparation

Dietary preparation is important to uncover colorectal carcinoma. The patient requires dietary restrictions for three days, as certain foods can give incorrect recordings (false positives and false negatives). This requires the patient to avoid:

- high fibre
- red meat
- raw vegetables
- raw fruit
- horseradish
- parsnips
- turnip
- melon,
- broccoli
- excess vitamin C (above 0.5 g/d)
- excess iron (above 1 g/d).

It is usual for asymptomatic patients to require three individual collections over a three-day period.

The Test

1. Wash and dry your hands and put on apron and gloves.
2. Check the expiry date on the test slide and developer bottle.
3. Remove the test slide from the kit and write the patient's details on the front section of the slide.
4. Open the flap of the slide and check that the test areas are cream-coloured. If they have a bluish tint, do not use the slide.
5. Use one end of your applicator stick and smear a pea-sized sample of faeces over oval I.
6. Use the other end of the applicator stick to take a second pea-sized sample of faeces from a different area of the sample and smear this over oval II.
7. Now close the front flap and turn the slide over and wait for a minimum of two minutes or a maximum of 14 days for the sample to react with the slide.
8. Open the back flap of the slide and apply two drops of the developer to each oval.
9. Time for exactly 60 seconds.
10. After 60 seconds, read the results from the ovals.
11. Place one drop of developer on to the control area.
12. For the test to be valid the POS (positive) areas must change to blue and the NEG (negative) areas must remain clear. If the control area does not do this, then repeat the test with a fresh slide.
13. A positive result is when there is any trace of blue colouring in either of the test areas. A negative result is when there is no blue colouring in either test area. Document and report your results. Figure 10.5 shows examples of positive and negative results.

Sources of Blood in the Faeces

- *Normal blood loss*: normal faecal blood loss is about 1–2 ml per day. The Hema-screen test detects blood amounts of 3–6 ml per day.

(a)

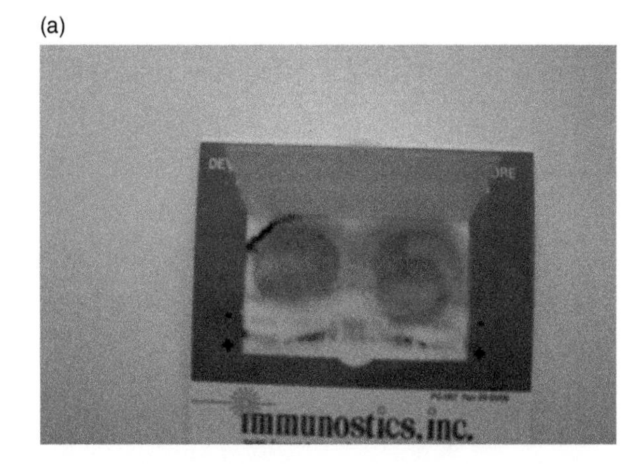

(b)

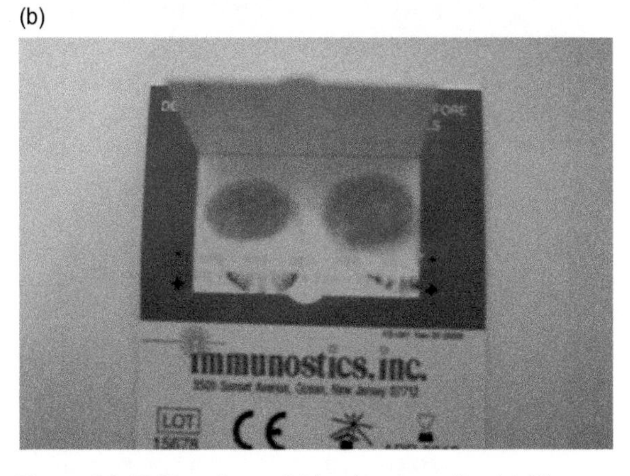

Figure 10.5 Faecal occult blood test results. (a) Blue present, meaning a positive result. (b) No blue present, which is a negative result.

- *Clinical conditions*: bowel and colon disease, tumours, ulcers (both stomach and intestines) and haemorrhoids.
- *Medication*: aspirin, indomethacin, corticosteroids, reserpine, phenylbutazone, etc.
- *Artefactual*: menstrual bleeding, dental work, blood from tester's hands.

Box 10.2 highlights the issues to be considered when checking blood in the faeces.

Box 10.2 Issues to Consider when Checking Blood in the Faeces

- If the patient is not clean, the sample may be contaminated and an incorrect result reported.
- Colorectal cancers can bleed intermittently and may require a change of diet and collections on three separate days to detect bleeding.
- Excessive vitamin C intake can give falsely negative results.
- The test slides should only be used on faecal samples, not any other type of fluid (pleural fluids, knee fluids, cerebral spinal fluid, etc.).
- Blood may be present due to menstruation. Allow three days before and three days after menstruation before faecal occult blood testing (GPs may suggest just two days if this test is performed at home).
- False positives may occur if large amounts of raw fruit, vegetables, fibre, horseradish, parsnips, turnips, melon, broccoli, or red meat are present in the diet.
- Iron-containing preparations may cause false-positive results to be seen, although a normal therapeutic dose (3 × 65 mg per day) should not interfere with the results. Iron may also turn the faeces black, thus masking the positive blue colour.

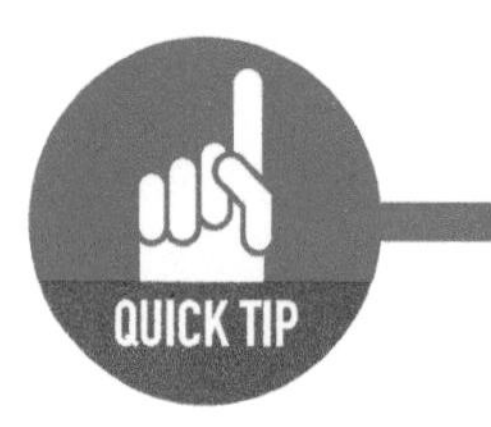

The recommended daily allowance for vitamin C varies. In the UK, it is 60 mg per day, although some countries, such as the United States, recommendations are much higher than this (3000 mg!).

If the test results are inconsistent with the patient's condition, retest with a fresh sample.

As with the urinalysis testing, it should be remembered that all patient samples are a potential infection risk and health and safety procedures must be adhered to, including disposal of used materials. One other consideration for the Hema-screen test is that the developer is flammable and should be kept well away from potential ignition sources.

BLOOD LANCING

Blood lancing is performed to obtain capillary blood samples. One reason to do it is to obtain a drop of blood to put on a slide for testing in a blood glucose monitor. This is the only way we can perform a blood glucose monitoring test.

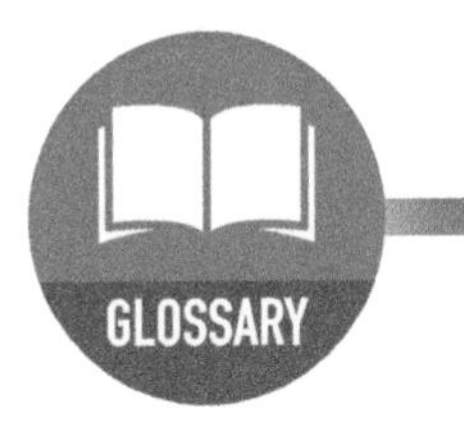

Phenylketonuria (PKU)
A very rare condition that can cause mental disability. The condition is treatable once diagnosed.

Blood lancing is also performed to obtain blood samples during a 'heel-prick test' on babies. This test can identify a range of conditions, such as sickle cell disease, cystic fibrosis, phenylketonuria and congenital hypothyroidism.

The device we look at in this chapter for the procedure is the Unistik® (Owen Mumford) blood lancet. There are four different types of Unistik lancets (Table 10.1), depending on gauge and patient.

Table 10.1 Unistik lancets.

Comfort	**Gauge: 28G** **Depth: 1.8mm** **To be used for blood glucose analysis**
Neonatal	**Gauge: 18G** **Depth: 1.8mm** **To be used for neonatal screening only**
Normal	**Gauge: 23G** **Depth: 1.8mm**
Extra	**Gauge: 21G** **Depth: 2.0mm** **To be used for haemoglobinometers only**

The Test

1. Wash and dry your hands and put on gloves and apron.
2. Clean the sampling site with soap and warm water. Do not use alcohol wipes, as they cool the site and harden the skin over time. Dry the collection site thoroughly.
3. Ensure that there is a good blood supply to the sampling site. This can be achieved by positioning the limb so that it is hanging down or by warming the sample site, or by getting the patient to exercise the limb.
4. Select the correct type of Unistik 3 lancet.
5. Rotate the cap until it comes free. This usually takes two or three rotations.
6. Remove the cap and discard it.
7. Position the Unistik 3 lancet so that it is within the correct sampling zones; that is, on the upper outer aspects of the fingers or on a baby's outer heel. Press down firmly.
8. Press the release button on the lancet.
9. After blood collection, use gauze and gentle pressure until the blood flow stops.

Blood sampling sites are the upper outer aspects of the fingers. Try to avoid the thumb and index finger. If repeat sampling is required, it is important to rotate the sampling site.

The sampling area for a baby is on the outer aspects of the side heel. Migration from this sampling zone on baby's heel will cause calcification of the heel and long-term problems with mobility for the baby.

The type of lancet used for blood lancing is designed to be less painful when lancing. You will notice that the end platform of the lancet has a circle of raised bumps (Figure 10.6). These activate the C nerve fibres in the skin. These fibres can gate the pain transmitted by the Aα and Aβ nerve fibres, which should reduce the pain felt by the patient.

Box 10.3 highlights issues to consider when using Unistik.

Box 10.3 Issues to Consider when using Unistik

- Make sure that you use the correct version of the Unistik 3.
- Always stay within the correct blood collection zones.

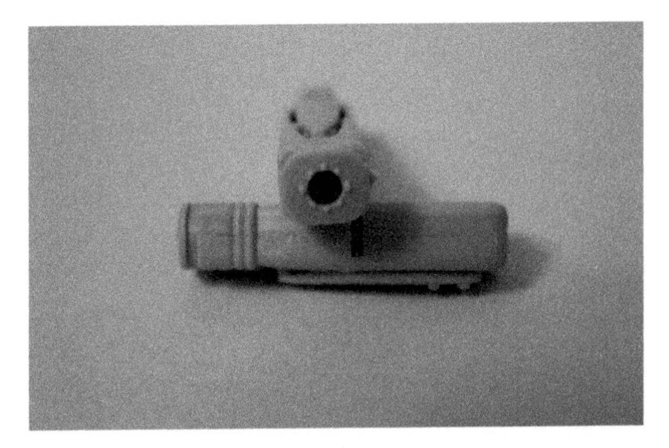

Figure 10.6 Raised circle of bumps on a blood lancet.

The lancet should be discarded into the nearest sharps container.

BLOOD GLUCOSE TESTING

There are many different devices on the market to monitor a patient's blood glucose level. This section describes the principles of blood glucose monitoring and does not focus on using any specific machine. You will, of course, need to be trained for the device your clinical area presently uses. These devices can be held in the hand or placed on large station ports.

The patient will first require to have one of their digits lanced to obtain the blood sample. Blood glucose monitoring is usually conducted on all patients during routine admission and on patients with diabetes.

Blood Glucose Levels

'Blood glucose' and 'blood sugar levels' are synonymous terms used to express the amount of glucose present in the blood, known as the plasma glucose level. Normal blood glucose levels vary throughout the day but tend to remain between 4 and 8 mmol/l, being lowest in the early morning and higher after meals. Ideal values may be:

- 4–7 mmol per litre before meals
- less than 10 mmol per litre 90 minutes after a meal
- around 8 mmol per litre at bedtime.

However, it should always be remembered that we are individuals and our 'norm' may vary from the 'ideal'. Also, in cardiopulmonary resuscitation a blood glucose reading of 4–10 mmol per litre is often the acceptable range.

People with diabetes may have more fluctuations in their blood glucose levels and may need to be monitored more closely. Table 10.2 shows the different types of diabetes.

Table 10.2 Different types of diabetes.

Type of diabetes	May also be known as	Information
Type 1 diabetes	Insulin-dependent diabetes mellitus (IDDM)	The body is unable to produce insulin. Usually starts in childhood or young adulthood. Treated with dietary control and insulin injections. Regular physical activity is recommended.
Type 2 diabetes	Non-insulin dependent diabetes mellitus (NIDDM)	The body does not produce enough insulin or this insulin does not work properly (insulin resistance). Tends to affect people as they get older, usually appearing after the age of 40 years, but it is increasingly being seen in younger people, especially if they are overweight or obese. Treated with diet and physical activity or by diet, physical activity and oral medication. May require insulin therapy as disease progresses.

Normal Blood Sugar Control: The Science Bit

The glucose that we ingest from sweet and starchy foods gets turned into energy. Insulin is a hormone manufactured by the pancreas; it regulates the amount of glucose in the blood. When levels of glucose in the body rise, such as just after eating a meal, the pancreas is triggered to release insulin, which then starts to stimulate the cells in the body to absorb the glucose. Without insulin, the glucose levels in the blood would just keep rising and cells in the body would be unable to use it for energy, resulting in extreme tiredness, as often experienced by those with untreated diabetes. Insulin also stimulates the liver to absorb some of the glucose and store any that is left over. The pancreas also manufactures another hormone called glucagon. When glucose levels in the blood are low, this hormone is released into the bloodstream and stimulates the liver to release the stored glucose, thus raising the glucose in the blood.

The Impact on the Individual

It has been estimated that there are more than 750 000 people in the UK with diabetes who do not know that they have the condition. The main symptoms are some or all of the following:

- increased thirst
- urinating more frequently: especially at night
- extreme tiredness
- weight loss
- genital itching
- regular episodes of thrush
- blurred vision.

Diabetes that is not controlled can cause many serious long-term health problems, such as damaged blood vessels, which in turn contributes to cardiovascular disease (such as hypertension, heart attack and stroke), kidney disease (nephropathy), eye disease (retinopathy) and nerve disease (neuropathy). Uncontrolled diabetes can also result in blindness and amputation.

People with diabetes who drive must inform the Driving and Vehicle Licencing Agency (DVLA) that they have diabetes.

Although there is no cure for diabetes, individuals with the condition should not be restricted from enjoying a full life. The organisation Diabetes UK works very hard at ending discrimination and ignorance for those with diabetes.

The Impact on the NHS

The NHS spends over 10% of its budget treating diabetes and this figure is set to rise. This is due to what has been described as an 'epidemic' in obesity in Western countries, resulting in huge increases in type 2 diabetes. Government scientists have predicted that over one-third of Britons can now be classed as obese.

Treatment

Individuals with type 1 diabetes require insulin therapy. This is administered via injection to replace insulin that the body is not producing. As insulin may be short, medium or long acting; some people may need to inject themselves up to three times a day with an insulin pen, just before meals.

Presently, insulin still needs to be given by injection and not by mouth, as the digestive juices and enzymes would destroy it before it is able to enter the bloodstream and be effective. New innovations are being developed, such as inhaled insulin formats and under-the-skin insulin-releasing rods.

Treatment for type 2 diabetes is first managed by lifestyle changes. If these are not effective, oral drug therapy will be required. As diabetes is a progressive disease, people with type 2 diabetes may require insulin eventually.

Everyone with diabetes should eat a diet that is low in fat, sugar and salt, and should maintain regular physical activity. This is because during exercise the level of glucose in the blood falls, resulting in insulin levels also falling. The aim is to maintain a steady blood glucose level.

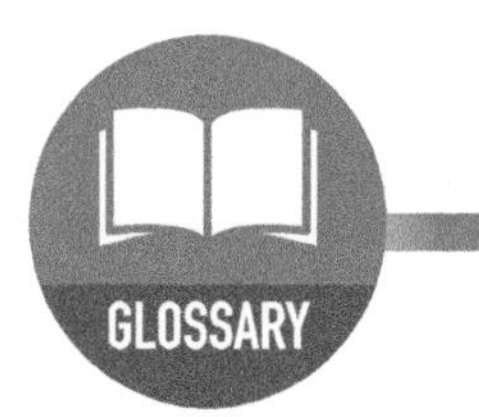

Hypo-glycaemia
When blood sugars go too low.
Hyper-glycaemia
When blood sugars go too high.

Monitoring

Monitoring the blood glucose level is a relatively quick and simple procedure, as long as it is conducted correctly. Whichever kit you use, you will need a measuring device, a test strip, a blood lancing device and a sharps box.

1. Wash your own hands prior to starting the test. Use warm soapy water. Dry thoroughly. Put on gloves and apron.
2. Wash the patient's hand prior to starting the test. Use sterile water. Dry thoroughly.
3. Do not use alcohol wipes as this will interfere with the test.
4. Prepare your machine. Check that the test strips have been correctly calibrated to the device (this will be displayed on the device screen).
5. Place the test strips in machine (this depends on which type of machine you are using).
6. Lance the patient's finger, aiming for a ladybird-sized drop of blood. Wipe off this first drop.
7. Gently squeeze the finger (not too hard as this may alter the test reading) to obtain another drop of blood.
8. Place this drop of blood on the test strip.
9. Read the results according to the manufacturer's instructions.
10. Document the results and act on any concerns.

Usually, if the result is less than 3.0 mmol/l or greater than 20 mmol/l, a medic will request that a venous sample be sent to the laboratory to confirm hypoglycaemia or hyperglycaemia, but this may vary according to the trust.

Sources of contamination include:

- newsprint (newspapers contain starch)
- residual sugars from soft drinks or foods
- the tester's own hands (if not wearing gloves).

TEST YOUR KNOWLEDGE

1 What do Combur 5 reagent strips test for?
2 How long can a sample of urine be left standing before it must be discarded and cannot be used for urinalysis?
3 Where should the Hema-screen developer be stored?
4 Where are the correct sampling zones for blood lancing?
5 What is hypoglycaemia?
6 When urinalysis testing, what do we need to be mindful of in relation to vegetarians?

KEY POINTS

- How to conduct an urinalysis test.
- How to undertake a faecal occult blood test.
- Correct procedures for blood lancing for blood glucose monitoring.
- Blood glucose testing.

USEFUL WEB RESOURCES

Lab Tests Online UK. Point of care testing: https://labtestsonline.org.uk/articles/point-care-testing

Science Direct. Point-of-care testing: https://www.sciencedirect.com/topics/medicine-and-dentistry/point-of-care-testing

Chapter 11

VENEPUNCTURE

LEARNING OUTCOMES

By the end of this chapter you will have an understanding of the theory and practice of performing the clinical skill of venepuncture.

WHAT IS VENEPUNCTURE?

The term venepuncture is exactly what the word suggests: entering a vein with a needle, by which we can obtain a sample of blood. It is one of the most commonly performed invasive procedures performed in the healthcare setting. Figure 11.1 shows this procedure being performed.

In the healthcare environment, there are many different makes of equipment for venepuncture: the BD Vacutainer® (BD, Franklin Lakes, NJ) system and the S-Monovette® (Sarstedt, Nümbrecht, Germany) system are just two. Whichever system is used, it must be one designed for the purpose: a needle and syringe *should not* be used generally, although it is accepted practice in many neonatal areas and for some medics.

The collection bottles are colour coded according to the blood test to be carried out and the additives contained in

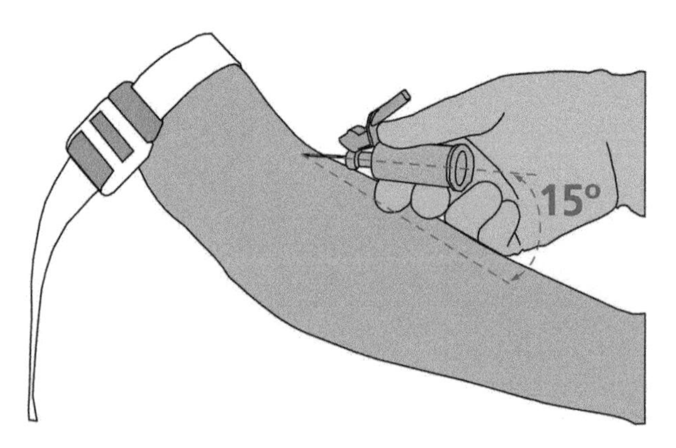

Figure 11.1 The venepuncture procedure. Source: Reproduced with kind permission from BD Diagnostics.

the tube (e.g. serum gel, heparin). Gloves should be worn when carrying out the venepuncture procedure, adhering as closely to possible to the aseptic technique (known as the aseptic non-touch technique or ANTT; see Chapter 1). It is also considered best practice for practitioners to check their hepatitis vaccine status to confirm that they are up to date with this immunisation.

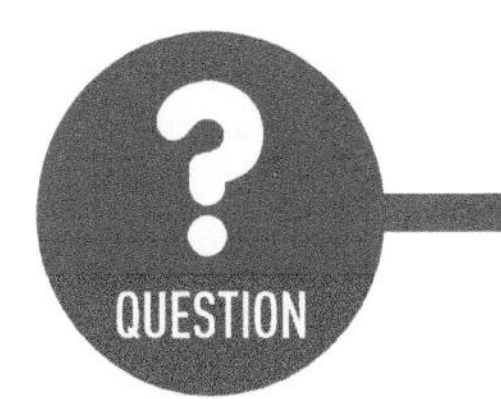

Question 11.1 What do you think are the five main reasons the clinical skill of venepuncture is performed?

The clinical skill of venepuncture is undertaken for five main reasons:

1. To obtain blood to rule out medical conditions (e.g. deep vein thrombosis)
2. To monitor levels of blood components (e.g. full blood count)
3. To obtain blood for diagnosis (e.g. troponin)
4. To prepare for a blood transfusion (e.g. crossmatch)
5. To monitor drug levels in the blood (e.g. warfarin).

To understand what these tests are, let's look at some of the common blood tests.

COMMON BLOOD TESTS

Venepuncture can be undertaken to obtain a blood sample for testing.

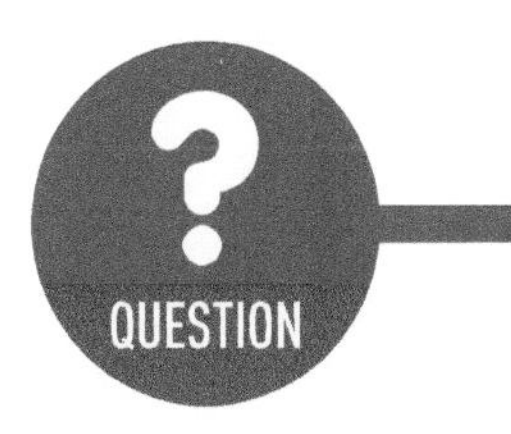

Question 11.2 Before we begin, can you name four common blood tests?

Full Blood Count

A full blood count is one of the most common blood tests and is usually carried out as part of a routine check. The haematology laboratory will often divide the full blood count (FBC) into five results:

1. **Red blood cell count:** erythrocytes are the most abundant cell type in the blood. By calculating their concentration it is possible to identify whether the patient is anaemic (low concentration) or polycythaemic (high concentration).
2. **Haemoglobin concentration:** haemoglobin is the oxygen-carrying component of erythrocytes. If the concentration is low, it is usually an indicator of anaemia.
3. **White cell count:** white blood cells, or leucocytes, form part of the body's defence against infections. They are normally found in low concentrations unless an infection is present, when their number increases.
4. **Differential blood count:** this identifies the concentrations of white blood cells, of which there are five types:
   - **a** neutrophils (comprising 50–70% of leucocytes)
   - **b** lymphocytes (20–40%)
   - **c** monocytes (3–8%)
   - **d** eosinophils (2–4%)
   - **e** basophils (0.5–1%).
5. **Platelet count:** an integral part of the clotting system, platelets basically plug the hole when bleeding occurs.

Erythrocyte Sedimentation Rate

The erythrocyte sedimentation rate (ESR) is the measurement of the erythrocyte settling rate in anticoagulated blood. Tissue destruction and inflammatory conditions can cause a raised ESR. This result can be very useful in assessing the degree of disease.

C-reactive Protein

C-reactive protein (CRP) has a similar function as the ESR and is used to monitor the acute phase response of many infections. These levels will rise dramatically in response to bacterial infection, trauma, tissue damage and inflammation.

Liver Function Test

A liver function test (LFT) comprises of a number of tests to allow detection of liver disease, placing liver disease into specific category and monitoring the progression of the disease.

Urea and Electrolytes

Urea and electrolytes (U&Es) measured in a blood serum sample allow monitoring of kidney and liver function. Urea is the waste product resulting from protein metabolism. Proteins are broken down by digestion into amino acids, which are then sent to the liver. The liver breaks them down further resulting in ammonia, which is toxic to the human body.

High urea levels could indicate:

- renal disease
- urinary obstruction
- shock
- congestive heart failure
- burns.

Low urea levels could indicate:

- liver failure
- pregnancy
- over-hydration
- starvation.

Electrolytes include:

- sodium
- potassium
- chloride
- bicarbonate
- creatinine.

Partial Thromboplastin Time

Partial thromboplastin time measures the plasma coagulation factors of the intrinsic pathway, derived from the reagents used in the test to initiate the reaction (activated partial thromboplastin activator, aPTT). The aPTT can be increased by:

- deficiencies of plasma proteins specific to the intrinsic pathway
- heparin
- degradation products
- pathological inhibitors
- severely overdosed warfarin patients.

Prothrombin Time

Prothrombin time (PT) assesses the activity of the extrinsic pathway of blood coagulation. It can be used to detect abnormalities in plasma coagulation. The time taken for the blood to clot when tissue factor and calcium are added is measured. Abnormalities are associated with:

- anticoagulants
- liver damage
- vitamin K deficiency
- overdoses of warfarin.

International Normalised Ratio

The international normalised ratio (INR) is a measurement of blood clotting time. The higher the INR, the longer it will take for your blood to clot. It was introduced by the World Health Organization to provide a common basis for interpretation of prothrombin time. INR is calculated from the patient's PT and a parameter called the International Sensitivity Index. This accounts for differences in manufacturers' standard samples so that INRs are comparable between laboratories.

Calcium

Calcium is the fifth most common element in the human body. Plasma calcium is necessary for maintaining a normal heart rhythm, the functioning of neurons and muscle contraction, and is involved in the coagulation of blood.

Low plasma calcium levels (hypocalcaemia) may indicate:

- low levels of parathyroid hormone
- vitamin D deficiency
- kidney damage
- certain bone diseases
- low calcium intake in the diet.

High plasma calcium levels (hypercalcaemia) may indicate:

- overdose of vitamin D
- increased levels of parathyroid hormone
- certain cancers
- high levels of calcium in the diet.

Cholesterol

Cholesterol is a major component of cell membranes; it is excreted in bile or metabolised in bile acids. High levels of cholesterol in the blood can cause severe problems to the arterial and venous systems, building up on vessels and causing inflammation, scarring and eventual blockage of the vessel.

Glucose

Glucose is a simple monosaccharide produced as a result of the digestion of starch and sucrose. The level of glucose in the body is highly regulated by the endocrine function of the pancreas. By monitoring the blood glucose level, it is possible to detect whether a patient has poor glucose level control. A high level (hyperglycaemia) may indicate diabetes.

D-Dimer

A D-dimer test may be ordered when someone has symptoms of deep vein thrombosis, such as leg pain or tenderness usually in one leg, leg swelling (oedema), discolouration of the leg.

Troponin

Troponin is a protein that is released into the bloodstream when the heart muscle is damaged. The troponin level provides a quick and accurate measure of any heart muscle damage.

POLICIES, PROCEDURES AND GUIDELINES

When undertaking the clinical skill of venepuncture, staff must have undertaken specialised training and had assessment for competency. Staff should also be familiar with their local policy for venepuncture, and other relevant policies and acts around:

- sharps handling and disposal
- informed consent
- Mental Capacity Act 2005
- handling and transportation of pathology specimens
- blood transfusion
- waste management.

VICARIOUS LIABILITY

It is important to work within your own boundaries, otherwise you may be breaking vicarious liability, which is a legal term defined as:

> the principle by which a practitioner's employer will take liability for the actions and omissions of the employee as long as they are acting within their job description and boundaries approved by the employer (Tilley and Watson, 2008).

KEEPING UPDATED

After attending a study session on venepuncture or having completed a recognised e-learning package to your area, certification and assessment documentation should be kept in a portfolio as evidence. As with all clinical skills, the skill of obtaining blood should be revisited on a regular basis to keep yourself updated. This may take the form of self-directed learning or by attending a clinical skills update session at your workplace.

EQUIPMENT USED FOR VENEPUNCTURE

The equipment used for obtaining the blood sample depends on the system you are using: this may be a bottle with a coloured top and needle or, if using the BD Vacutainer system, a blood collection holder, bottle and needle (Figure 11.2). Some of the newer systems now have the needle and holder integrated, into which the blood bottle is pushed into and punctured. The needle is then covered with a plastic cuff at the end of the procedure as a safety measure to cut down on sharps injuries (Figure 11.3).

WRITTEN REQUESTS

In the hospital setting, a request form will need to be completed by a nurse practitioner or medic, requesting the blood sample to be obtained. Requests for blood transfusions will also need to be completed prior to collecting the sample (see Chapter 14). An example of one of these request forms can be seen in Figure 11.4.

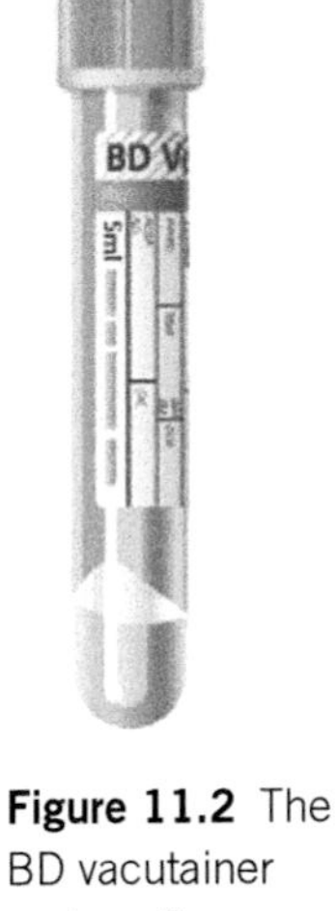

Figure 11.2 The BD vacutainer system. Source: Reproduced with kind permission from BD Diagnostics.

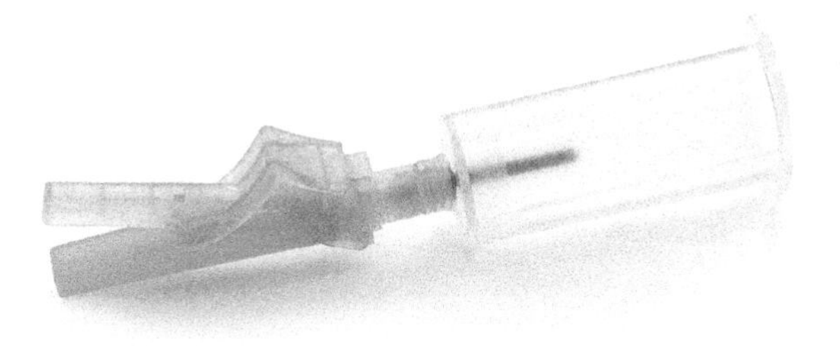

Figure 11.3 A safety-cuffed venepuncture system. Source: Reproduced with kind permission from BD Diagnostics.

NORTH BRISTOL NHS TRUST
DEPARTMENT OF BLOOD TRANSFUSION

NHS No. / Hospital No. including Hospital prefix

Surname Please place approved Addressograph in this area

Forename

D.O.B. D D M M Y Y Y Y — Sex (M/F) — Patient Type NHS PP Cat II

Patients Address inc. Post Code

Consultat / GP Code — Location Code

Clinical Details / Therapy

Requesting Doctor .... Bleep No. ....
Signature .... Date & Time ....

Sample Collection
I confirm that I have taken the blood sample for this request in accordance with the NBT Policy, (Summary overleaf) and labelled in the presence of the patient. I have confirmed the patients identity both verbally and with the wristband where available.
Name .... Signature ....
Date and Time ..../............/........... ....:...........

Group and Hold

X-Match
Product — No of Units
Date & Time required
D D M M Y Y H H M M
Patient requires Special Blood Products? Y / N
If Yes Give Details ....

Foetal Leak

Other Requests ....

Previously Transfused? (Y/N) ....
When? ....
Any reactions? ....
Blood Group ....
Any irregular antibodies? ....
Most recent Hb ....

For Laboratory Use			Inoculation Risk? YES ☐	NO ☐			
				RT	IAG	Time	Initial
ABO	D	Ab Screen					

Frenchay Hospital, Telephone Bristol 0117 340 2780
Southmead Hospital, Telephone Bristol 0117 323 5630

Figure 11.4 Blood sample request form for blood transfusion. Source: Permission to reproduce this image is granted by North Bristol NHS Trust and University Hospitals Bristol NHS Foundation Trust.

AVAILABLE VEINS

Blood samples are ideally obtained from the median cubital vein across the antecubital fossa (where the arm bends). It is important that health carers performing the clinical skill of venepuncture have an understanding of this basic anatomy, in order not to stab an artery with the needle, so you may wish to look up the blood vessels in the arm.

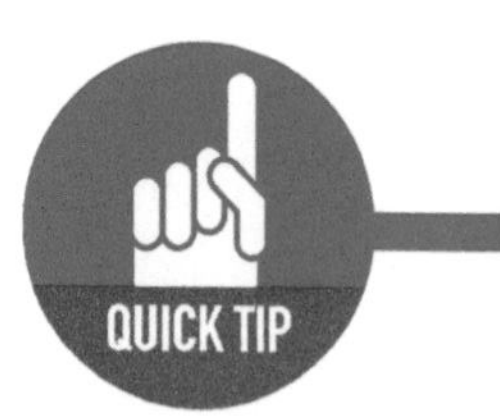

Arteries are the same side as the little finger. Go up the arm from the little finger, feel for a pulse in the antecubital fossa and then go to the opposite side along this crease until you feel the blood vessel with no pulse. Voila: a vein!

The antecubital fossa is the approved site for venepuncture because:

- it is able to tolerate repeat samples
- it is the most stable vein
- it is one of the larger veins
- it is close to the surface of the body
- it is said to be the least sensitive area.

Medics and other specialist health carers sometimes obtain blood samples from the groin, feet or neck, but this is certainly not routine. Obtaining a sample from the feet may cause the patient to experience an air embolism or other complication, such as necrosis in patients with diabetes.

Vein Anatomy

Veins have three layers. They also contain valves, which help, with muscle movement, to shunt the blood back towards the heart. Connective tissue helps to keep the veins in place. As we get older, there may be a loss of connective tissue, and the vessels can become quite mobile and will require some traction (downwards pulling) to be stabilised and straightened. As valves are sited all along the veins, we may inadvertently hit one, which will cause the patient some pain. If this happens then remove the needle and dispose of it, apologise to the patient and explain what has happened and that the vein will repair itself.

The Ideal Vein

Veins do not have a pulse and will refill when depressed. The vein needs to be soft and bouncy, and ideally it should be well supported by subcutaneous tissue. Sometimes the vein may be visible. It is always considered good practice to ask the patient's preference for which arm to use, and they may also know which arm is better for giving blood.

The Poor Vein

When selecting the vein for venepuncture we should try to avoid mobile, hard and inflamed or painful veins. Also stay away from bruised or infected areas. We should avoid areas where intravenous fluids or medication are being transfused, and should opt for the opposite arm.

Extra skill will be required by the health carer for patients with damaged veins, such as intravenous drug abusers.

Vein Selection

Prior to selecting the vein for venepuncture we will need to know the clinical status of our patient. For example, if a patient (male or female) has undergone breast surgery, they may be experiencing lymphoedema (lymph drainage problems), so we will need to obtain our sample from the other, non-affected arm. If this patient has undergone a double mastectomy, and for patients who have peripherally shut down, it is more usual for medics or specialised staff to perform the venepuncture.

In addition, patients on medication that slows down the clotting cascade will require more pressure on the puncture site, as the bleeding will take longer to stop when the needle is removed from the vein. It is not correct to say that drugs such as heparin, aspirin and warfarin 'thin the blood': it is the clotting factor that is affected.

It is important to involve the patient in the venepuncture procedure and to try to put them at their ease and gain their cooperation. Listen to the patient: have they had this procedure performed previously? Ask 'How was it for you?' In this way, we are gathering information on the patient and the way in which we have performed the technique (to be forewarned is to be forearmed!).

It is very difficult to obtain a blood sample from a patient who is dehydrated and from those with difficult-to-locate veins (such as patients with obesity), so it is important to know your limitations and not attempt the procedure if you do not have the competence. It is usual to only make two attempts at venepuncture, or three in an emergency.

SKIN CLEANING

The venepuncture site should be cleaned thoroughly with a cleaning agent, such as with a 70% isopropyl alcohol/2% chlorhexidine wipe (e.g. a Clinell® swab) or a 70% isopropyl alcohol wipe (e.g. Steret®). It must then be left to dry. Povidone iodine 10% should be used as an alternative if the patient is sensitive to chlorhexidine. It is recommended that the site is not repalpated after cleansing, although this may be necessary if the patient's vein is very difficult to find.

ORDER OF DRAW

The order of draw is the order in which the blood samples should be collected. Each of the coloured-topped bottles contain chemicals to prevent clotting of the sample, and some of these chemicals may dribble out and contaminate the next sample.

Figure 11.5 shows an example of the order of draw, but it is important to establish the order of draw for the area in which you are collecting samples and for the system of venepuncture that you are using.

Sodium Citrate Tubes

- Sodium citrate tubes are used to test clotting and in monitoring anticoagulant therapy (e.g. warfarin).
- Usually, this is the first bottle to be filled.
- Fill until the vacuum is exhausted.
- You must fill above the frosted line, as pathology laboratories often have to reject samples unless they are filled to this level (Figure 11.6).
- If using a butterfly, discard the first citrate tube and use another.

Once the blood sample is in the tube, you will need to gently invert the sample (do not shake vigorously). The number of times the bottle needs to be inverted depends on the sample, either 3–4 times, 5–6 times or 8–10 times. Looking at the order of draw chart, you can see that the sodium citrate tubes requires three to four inversions to mix the blood sample and preserving fluid with this make of tube.

LABELLING THE TUBES

Many sampling errors are made through the venepuncture sample not being labelled at the bedside. It is therefore good practice to label the tubes as soon as the sample has

BD Vacutainer®

BD Diagnostics - Preanalytical Systems

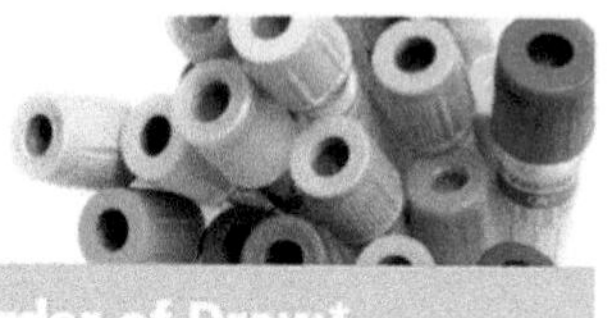

Tube Guide & Recommended Order of Draw*

* Clinical and Laboratory Standards Institute (Formerly NCCLS) Guidelines H3-A6, 6th Edition

North Bristol NHS Trust

Emergency Department, Acute Assessment Unit, ICU

Blood samples must be taken in the following order:

	Cap Colour	Additive	Tests	Special Instructions
1		Blood Culture	Aerobic followed by Anaerobic - if insufficient blood for both culture bottles, use Aerobic bottle only.	
2		Sodium Citrate	Clotting studies, INR, Heparin monitoring, Warfarin monitoring, D-Dimer.	Tube MUST be filled to the full draw volume. Mix 3-4 Times
3		SST™ II	Serum electrophoresis, lithium, Antibiotic assays, Immunology, serology.	Mix 5-6 Times
4		PST™ II	U&Es, LFT, Calcium, Lipids, Thyroid function test, CRP, Amylase, Magnesium, Vitamin B12, Folate, Ferritin.	Mix 8-10 Times
5		EDTA	Full blood count, plasma viscosity, immunosuppressants, Haemoglobin A1c, Parathyroid hormone, Sickle cell & thalassaemia, Malaria screens, ammonia.	Mix 8-10 Times
6		EDTA	Transfusion samples (Group & save, cross match, antenatal).	Mix 8-10 Times
7		Fluoride Oxalate	Glucose, Lactate, Ethanol.	Mix 8-10 Times
8		Trace Element	Zinc, Selenium, Aluminium, Copper, etc.	Mix 8-10 Times

For further copies of this guide and questions regarding specific tests, please contact the main Pathology Laboratory.

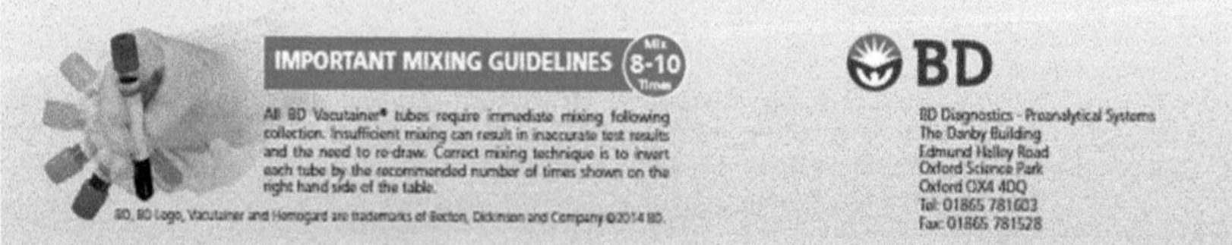

Figure 11.5 BD order of draw chart. Source: Reproduced with kind permission from BD Diagnostics.

been taken, and not to get distracted. Patients should have their identity bands checked against the documentation to establish that the correct patient is being venepunctured. The patient should also be asked to verbally state their name and date of birth, if possible.

Community situations have their own safety measures in place. For instance, care homes often have residents' pictures on the bedroom doors and, in health centres, patients attend scheduled appointments.

Any biohazard specimens should be well labelled and are usually double-bagged.

Figure 11.6 Sodium citrate tube.

POTASSIUM AND CALCIUM

When obtaining potassium or calcium samples a tourniquet should not be used. This is because a tourniquet slows the movement of blood and alters the chemicals obtained in the sample, showing higher readings. If a tourniquet is used, then it is usual to insert the needle into the vein, remove the tourniquet and wait for approximately one minute before obtaining the blood sample. The pathology laboratory should then be informed that a tourniquet was used.

PAEDIATRICS

Special precautions apply in children's nursing and special care baby units and neonatal intensive care units (NICU). In the NICU of many NHS trusts, no student doctors, healthcare assistants or radiographers may undertake venepuncture. Tourniquets are also not used in NICU. It is also quite common to see samples obtained using a needle and syringe instead of the fit-for-purpose equipment.

For infants weighing less than 1.5 kg or those aged less than 30 weeks, 0.05% chlorhexidine must be used. For infants weighing more than 1.5 kg or aged more than 30 weeks 0.5% chlorhexidine must be used.

PROBLEMS ASSOCIATED WITH VENEPUNCTURE

The main problems associated with venepuncture, apart from not being able to locate the vein in the first place, are:

- haematoma/bruising
- excessive pain
- needlestick injury
- fainting
- nerve damage
- infection
- hardening of the veins
- haemorrhage
- blood spillage
- arterial stab (i.e. stabbing an artery instead of the intended vein)
- embolism (air getting into bodily system).

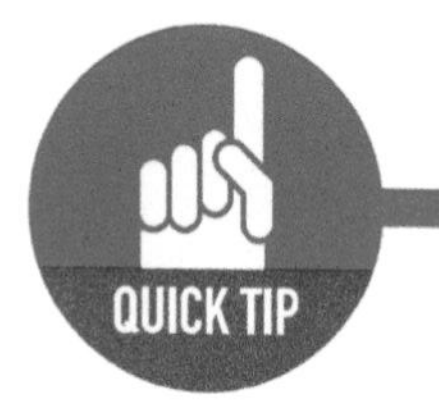

Don't panic if you do stab an artery. *Call for help,* put pressure on the site and reassure your patient.

Needlestick Injury

If you inadvertently stab yourself with a used needle you will need to:

1. Encourage the wound to bleed by squeezing.
2. Wash it thoroughly with running water.
3. Cover the wound with a waterproof dressing.
4. Call your local needlestick injury hotline and/or occupational health to report the injury.
5. Inform your manager/mentor and complete an accident form.

USING A TOURNIQUET

Placing a tourniquet approximately 10 cm above the intended puncture site creates stasis of the blood (i.e. slows down the blood flow). Tourniquets come in different designs and it is important to adhere to infection control principles and ideally use single-use tourniquets only to minimise spread of infection. Figure 10.6 shows a tourniquet in place.

Two fingers are placed under the tourniquet when tying or buckling up, to create the right amount of stasis, and so as not to cause pinching of the skin. Always check whether the tourniquet contains latex to protect your latex-sensitive patients (Figure 11.7).

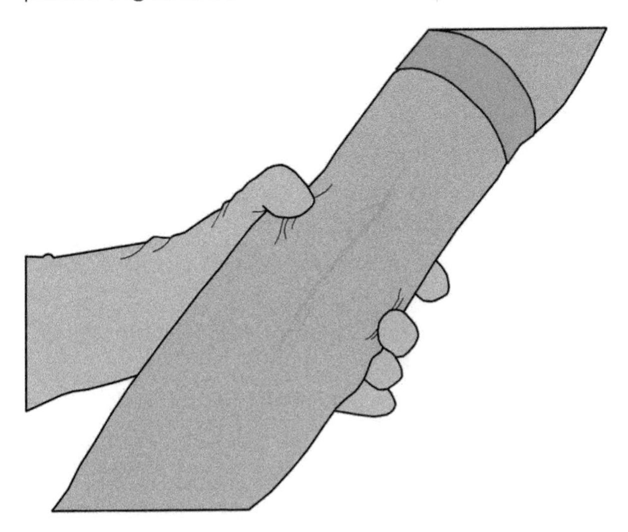

Figure 11.7 A tourniquet in place to create stasis of blood flow. Source: Reproduced with kind permission from BD Diagnostics.

The tourniquet should be moved as soon as possible; if it is kept on too long it may cause nerve damage. Blood pressure cuffs can also be used, up to the pressure of approximately 80 mmHg.

Catheter tubes and gloves must never be used as a tourniquet, as this is not what they were designed for! Squeezing the area with two hands is also not best practice.

GUIDELINES FOR THE VENEPUNCTURE PROCEDURE

Equipment needed	
Gloves (and plastic apron if contamination is unavoidable or patient is an infection risk) Cleaning agent: a 70% isopropyl alcohol/2% chlorhexidine wipe (e.g. a Clinell swab; 2% chlorhexidine is for adults: use 0.05% for infants weighing less than 1.5 kg and 0.5% for those more than 1.5 kg), a 70% isopropyl alcohol wipe (e.g. Steret) or povidone iodine 10% (if the patient is sensitive to chlorhexidine) Needle tubes Swabs Tourniquet (preferably disposable) Plastic sharps tray Plaster (if appropriate) Sharps box	
Procedure	
1	Explain the procedure to the patient, gaining valid consent.
2	Check that the identity of the patient matches the details on the request form or electronic register.
3	Gather equipment together on a plastic tray with the sharps bin and take to the bedside.
4	Assist the patient into an appropriate position to allow access to the limb for venepuncture.
5	Arrange the limb so that the patient is comfortable.
6	Apply the tourniquet, assess and select the appropriate vein and release the tourniquet.
7	Put on the plastic apron. Wash your hands using soap and water and the six-step hand-decontamination technique.
8	Open the outer plastic packaging and prepare equipment.
9	Put on the gloves.
10	Clean the patient's skin and the selected vein thoroughly. Allow to dry for 30 seconds. Do not repalpate the vein or touch the skin afterwards.
11	Reapply the tourniquet.
12	Remove the needle's sheath and inspect the needle for any faults.
13	Anchor the vein by applying manual traction on the skin a few centimetres below the proposed site of insertion.

14	**Ensure that the needle is in the bevel-up position and insert it through the skin at the selected angle according to the depth of the vein. Forewarn the patient that the vein is about to be punctured by stating 'sharp scratch'.**
15	**Reduce the angle of descent of the needle as soon as the vein has been punctured.**
16	**Pull back the plunger or leave until the required amount of blood is obtained by vacuum, depending on system being used.**
17	**Remove the first tube while keeping the needle still; apply any further tubes in accordance with the order of draw.**
18	**When all required samples are obtained, release the tourniquet.**
19	**Remove the needle, but do not apply pressure until the needle has been fully removed.**
20	**Apply digital pressure directly over the puncture site, using the swab.**
21	**Dispose of the needle into sharps container.**
22	**Gently the invert tubes.**
23	**Label the tubes with all relevant details.**
24	**Observe the site for signs of swelling or leakage and ask the patient if any discomfort or pain is felt.**
25	**Apply a dressing, if appropriate.**
26	**Discard waste in appropriate waste bins.**
27	**Remove gloves and apron, and wash hands.**
28	**Document date, time, site and reason for venepuncture in patient's record and send off the sample(s).**

Arterial Blood Gas

Undertaking an arterial blood gas sample is a very specialised clinical skill, requiring specialised training and are often referred to as an ABG. The needle is inserted at 30-degrees to the skin at the point of maximum pulsation of the radial artery. The needle is advanced until the arterial blood is sucked up into the syringe (via arterial pressure). The blood is then decanted into the tube via the bung in the tube. Most ABGs are collected today in all-in-one devices, negating the need to transfer the sample via the bung and the high possibility of sustaining a needle-stick injury. These are called blood transfer devices. ABGs are used to test for:

- pH – the acid/base balance of the arterial blood
- PCO_2 – how much carbon dioxide is in the blood
- PO_2 – how much oxygen is being concentrated in the blood
- HCO_3 – bicarbonate levels may indicate kidney function issues
- O_2 – how much oxygen is available for the tissues of the body.

TEST YOUR KNOWLEDGE

1. What is the maximum time that practitioners undertaking venepuncture are advised that tourniquets can stay in place?
2. Why should patients not clench their fists too hard and repeatedly (to bring up the veins) during venepuncture?
3. In relation to venepuncture, what is the order of draw?
4. At what age are individuals presumed to be able to give consent?
5. Practitioners undertaking venepuncture are advised by occupational health to have been immunised against what?
6. Before venepuncture is attempted, what must be obtained from the patient?
7. If a blood sample is ascertained to monitor drug levels, what must be recorded?
8. What is a differential blood count test?
9. What are the five types of white blood cells?
10. A sodium citrate tube type, as in order of draw, is used for what type of blood testing?

KEY POINTS

- Rationale for the venepuncture procedure.
- Common blood tests.
- Vein selection for venepuncture.
- Order of draw.
- Problems associated with venepuncture.
- The venepuncture procedure.

USEFUL WEB RESOURCES

BD. Specimen collection: https://www.bd.com/en-us/offerings/capabilities/specimen-collection

Geeky Medics. Venepuncture OSCE guide: https://geekymedics.com/venepuncture-how-to-take-blood

REFERENCE

Tilley, S. and Watson, R. (2008). *Accountability in Nursing and Midwifery*, 2e. Oxford: Blackwell Science.

Chapter 12

PERIPHERAL CANNULATION

Clinical Skills for Nurses, Second Edition. Claire Boyd.

LEARNING OUTCOMES

By the end of this chapter you will have an understanding of the theory and practice of performing the clinical skill of cannulation.

Peripheral venous cannulation is when a plastic or metal tube is inserted into a peripheral vein for intravenous (IV) drug therapy, fluid and electrolyte replacement or the transfusion of blood products. A further indication is for the administration of dyes and contrast media during clinical investigations. Some acute areas also insert a device for prophylactic reasons, 'just in case'.

The device used is a peripheral venous catheter (PVC), commonly referred to as a cannula. These devices come in different colour-coded sizes (known as the gauge size) and many different styles, depending on manufacturer. Figure 12.1 shows a typical PVC device. Blood samples can be obtained from this type of PVC, but usually only immediately after it has been inserted. However, if a patient has very poor veins and a blood sample cannot be obtained from any other site it is usually permitted, but you will need to check that this is accepted practice in your area. In this

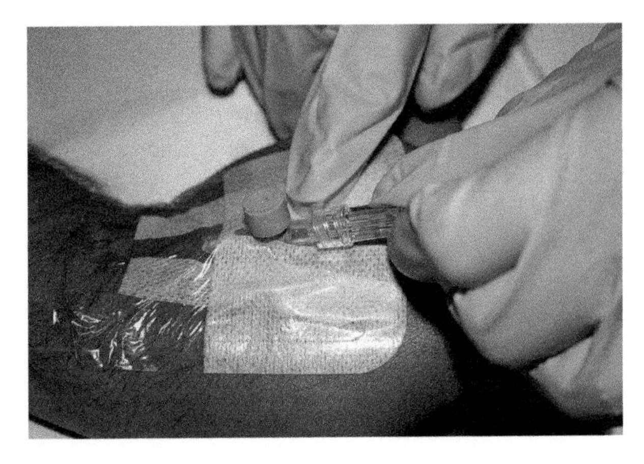

Figure 12.1 A peripheral venous catheter device.

case, the first 5 ml of blood will need to be discarded and the PVC flushed after the procedure.

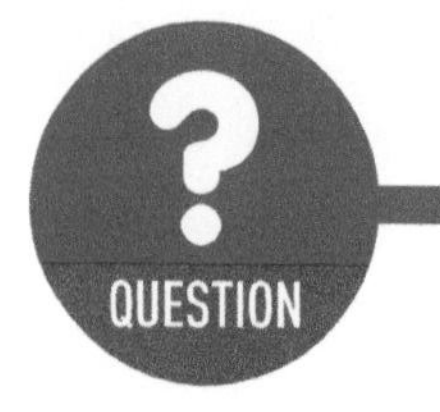

Question 12.1 For what reasons would you need to insert a PVC device? List five.

SELECTION OF AN APPROPRIATE CANNULA

A PVC must never totally occlude a vein, so the smallest cannula should be selected. However, if the patient is critically ill and the situation is an emergency, for example during hypovolaemic shock, this rule does not apply. Then we insert a larger device to 'push the fluids' into the patient's system as quickly as possible for rapid treatment.

We also need to think about the intended infusate and at what speed this fluid needs to 'go through'. This will have a bearing on our cannula choice.

A PVC device should usually be replaced after 72 hours (3 days), but should be flushed, usually with 0.9% sodium chloride every 4–6 hours (see section on Flushing).

Traditionally, a green cannula (18 gauge) was used to infuse blood as it was thought that a smaller gauge would damage the red blood cells. Most bags of blood are between 300 and 400 ml and should be administered within three to four hours. We can see from Table 12.1 that, in one hour, we can infuse up to 2700 ml (or 2.7 l) of blood via a green cannula (18 gauge or 18 G). Even in paediatrics we can run through 500 ml of blood via a yellow (24 gauge) and purple (26 gauge) cannula with this make of cannula. Note that the colour of the gauge sizes of other manufacturers may vary.

It is best practice to use intradermal local anaesthesia on small children and for adults when inserting an 18-gauge cannula or larger. If local anaesthetic is necessary, this should be applied 30–60 minutes prior to the cannulation.

Table 12.1 Cannula selection.

Colour	Common applications	Size gauge (G)	Approximate flow rate (l/hour)		
			Crystalloid	Plasma	Blood
Orange	Used in theatres or emergency for rapid transfusion of blood or viscous fluids	14	16.2	13.5	10.3
Grey	Used in theatres or emergency for rapid transfusion of blood or viscous fluids	16	10.8	9.4	7.1
White	Blood transfusions, rapid infusion of large volumes of viscous liquids	17	7.5	6.5	4.6
Green	Blood transfusions, parenteral nutrition, stem-cell harvesting and cell separation, large volumes of fluids	18	4.8	4.1	2.7
Pink	Blood transfusions, large volumes of fluids, diagnostic procedures (e.g. injection of contrast media)	20	3.2	2.9	1.9
Blue	Blood transfusions, most medications, and fluids	22	1.9	1.7	1.1
Yellow	Medications, short-term infusions, fragile veins, paediatrics, neonates or oncology patients undergoing chemotherapy	24	0.8	0.7	0.5
Purple	Neonatal	26	0.8	0.7	0.5

Source: Reproduced with kind permission of BD Diagnostics.

THE PERIPHERAL VENOUS CATHETER DEVICE

The cannula comes in three parts. Before using it, we need to check the packaging, which will tell us whether the device is latex-free and the fact that it is single use.

This packaging will also show us the gauge size, lot number and expiry date, as well as how many millilitres per minute can be infused through the device.

APPROVED SITE

It is usual to site a cannula on the back of the hand and then work your way up to the antecubital fossa (see Chapter 11). Doctors and some specialist nurses may cannulate in the legs and feet, but this is more problematic, as there is more chance of causing an air embolism at these sites, so nurses are generally not permitted to use them. In addition, patients with diabetes may experience more complications in the leg and feet, due to the small-fibre neuropathic damage that this disease causes.

Points of flexion should be avoided and the cannula secured with an appropriate dressing to avoid movement of the device.

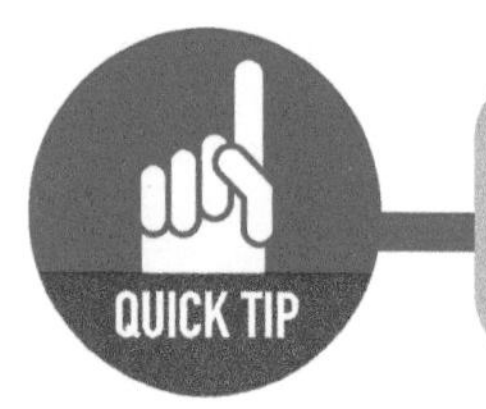

Always take your time selecting the appropriate site for insertion – never rush this part of the process.

VEIN SELECTION

Vein selection is by the same procedures as described for venepuncture (see Chapter 11), remembering to ask whether our patient has had this procedure before; in other words, involving them in the process.

Mobile veins on the back of the hands can be difficult to cannulate. In this case, we need to add a little traction, meaning that the vein should be pulled taut. It is for this reason that it is always best to practice your technique on patients who are a little easier to cannulate until you become more experienced.

The following areas should be avoided:

- The arm of patient who has undergone a mastectomy and/or axillary node dissection or radiotherapy.
- Limbs with fistulae or awaiting fistula formation.
- The affected side of a patient who has had a stroke.
- Limbs with fractures.
- Small, visible but impalpable veins.
- Veins on the palm side of the hands.
- Median cubital veins.
- Limbs affected by lymph node dissection or radiotherapy.
- Veins that feel hard and sclerosed.
- Areas of joint flexion.
- Veins in close proximity to arteries/arterial lines.
- Veins in upper arms.
- Veins in lower limbs.
- Previously cannulated veins.

NUMBER OF ATTEMPTS

It is usual to allow only two attempts when trying to insert a cannula. It is then best to ask someone else to cannulate the patient. Of course, in an emergency or if someone has very difficult veins, more than two attempts are often permitted.

SKIN PREPARATION

The site of cannulation should be cleaned thoroughly using a cleaning agent, such as 70% isopropyl alcohol/2% chlorhexidine wipe (e.g. a Clinell® swab) or a 70% isopropyl alcohol wipe. This should be left to dry for 30 seconds before proceeding. For patients sensitive to chlorhexidine, povidone iodine 10% should be used as an alternative. If injecting radiopharmaceuticals, 70% isopropyl alcohol is generally used to clean the skin. For neonates, skin cleaning may be as in Table 12.2, but again check with your own policies and procedures:

Table 12.2 Neonatal skin cleaning.

Age (weeks + days) and/or weight	Cleaning agent
<27+0 and/or ≥ 1 kg	Within first week of life: aqueous chlorhexidine 0.05%, chlorhexidine gluconate
	After the first week of life: chlorhexidine gluconate solution 0.5% in 70% alcohol
<27 +0 and/or >1kg at birth	Within first week of life: chlorhexidine gluconate solution 0.5% in 70% alcohol
All other babies	Chlorhexidine gluconate 4%

ASEPTIC NON-TOUCH TECHNIQUE

Apron and gloves should be worn during the procedure. If a patient is having IV fluids administered and the set-up needs to be disconnected when going to x-ray or elsewhere, a bung should be used to cover the administration port on the device and the line disconnected. A new line should be set up on the patient's return.

FLUSHING

A PVC device should be flushed, usually with 0.9% sodium chloride, every four to six hours. The procedure for this technique is called the **push–pause technique**. Draw up the flush and administer it by injecting approximately 1 ml, then stop, then push in another 1 ml and stop again. Continue with this process until the flush has been administered in full. The rationale for this procedure is to create many different episodes of turbulence to stop any build-up of clotted blood at the end of the cannula. When flushing, you should feel no/little resistance; it should go in like a hot knife through butter (or any other preferred spread)!

Neonates tend to have 0.5 ml flushes, before, between and after medication using the 10 ml syringe.

Nothing smaller than a 10 ml syringe should be used to flush a cannula, ideally with 10 ml of fluid. With smaller syringes, too much pressure may be applied to the vein. Prior to a flush the hub of the cannula should be cleaned, usually with the same substance we use to clean the skin, such as an alcohol wipe; this is known as 'scrubbing the hub'.

ATTACHMENTS

Most clinical areas use a long line (single or double), often called a microclave, which is primed with saline before use and then attached to the cannula. This line is where medications and flushes are administered instead of the hub of the cannula. These lines are used for infection control purposes (as any bugs have further to travel to the blood stream) and are for patient comfort. As stated, these lines must be primed (filled with saline) prior to attachment to the cannula to avoid pushing just air (in the line) into the patient's vein.

FIXATIONS AND DRESSINGS

The cannula should be secured with sterile, semi-permeable dressings that are transparent at the cannula entry site, so that we can view the site for any signs of infection. Dressings should always be changed when damp, soiled or loose. A dressing may not be required if the cannula is to be in for a very short time, such as 15 minutes.

A secondary fixation or dressing may be necessary, but should only be used if the patient is likely to knock the cannula out of place. The recommended secondary fixation in adults tends to be a two-way stretch tubular bandage (e.g.Tubifast®, but not Tubigrip® compression bandages). The bandage must be loose enough to allow free flow of blood around the limb, but tight enough to do its job (i.e. protect the cannula).

Bandages should only be used when there is no alternative available or where the patient is at risk of removing the cannula if it is not firmly secured (e.g. babies, children or confused patients). This secondary fixation/dressing should be removed and the cannulation site inspected each time the cannula is used or visually inspected.

DOCUMENTATION

Records must be kept of who inserted the device, where on the body it was and the date on which it was performed. The cannulation site should be inspected every shift and information recorded on the care plan.

All cannula sites should be covered by a transparent dressing so that the site can be inspected for any sign of phlebitis. This visual inspection is often called a VIP (for visual inspection of phlebitis) and a score is given to the site area. Figure 12.2 shows a typical cannulation care plan. We can see that for a score of two and above we should resite the cannula.

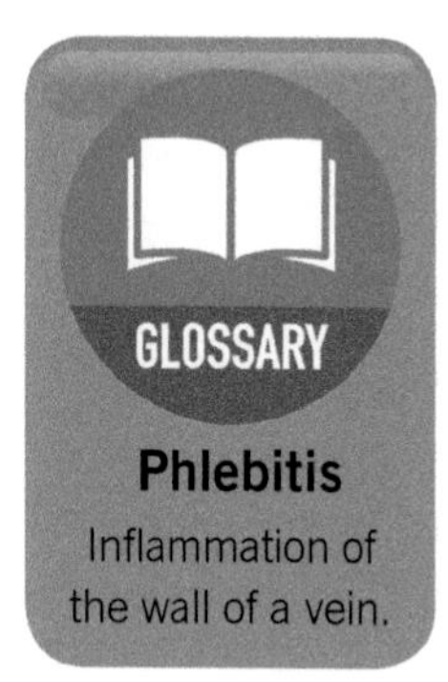

Phlebitis

Inflammation of the wall of a vein.

PROBLEMS ASSOCIATED WITH CANNULATION

The same problems apply to cannulation as venepuncture, namely infection, pain and nerve damage. Phlebitis is also a potential problem when performing this procedure. It can be caused by:

- infection: causing inflammation of the vein
- the cannula rubbing and irritating the lining of the vein (tunica intima): mechanical phlebitis
- the drug being infused, such as strongly alkaline, acidic, or hypertonic drugs: chemical phlebitis.

To minimise the incidences of such problems occurring, we can troubleshoot:

- Infection: ensure that an aseptic non-touch technique is used during insertion and assessment of the PVC.
- Mechanical phlebitis: ensure that the cannula is secured using the correct method for the dressing.

North Bristol 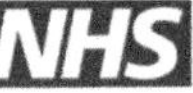
NHS Trust

Peripheral Cannulae Care Plan			
Name		Date of Birth	
Hospital Number		Department	
	Cannula 1	Cannula 2	Cannula 3
Location of Cannula			
Date of Insertion			
Time of Insertion			
Location of Insertion			
Insert by (Print Name)			
Reason for Cannulation			
Size/Colour of Cannula			
Date of Removal			
Time of Removal			
Removed by (Print Name)			

Visual Infusion Phlebitis (VIP) Score (adopted from Andrew Jackson's VIP score)		
Signs		**Actions**
Intravenous (IV) site appears healthy	0	No sign of phlebitis Observe cannula
Slight pain near IV site or Slight redness near IV site	1	Possible first sign of phlebitis Observe cannula
Two of the following: Pain near IV site Erythema Swelling	2	Early stage of phlebitis Resite cannula
Pain along path of cannula Erythema and Induration	3	Medium stage of phlebitis Resite cannula Consider treatment
All of the following is evident and extensive: Pain along path of cannula Erythema Induration Palpable venous cord	4	Advanced stage of phlebitis or start of thrombophlebitis Resite cannula Consider treatment
All of the following is evident and extensive: Pain along path of cannula Erythema Induration Palpable venous cord Pyrexia	5	Advanced stage of thrombophlebitis Initiate treatment Resite cannula

Figure 12.2 Peripheral cannula care plan. Source: Reproduced with permission from North Bristol NHS Trust and University Hospitals Bristol NHS Foundation Trust.

- Chemical phlebitis: dilutie medications as per manufacturers recommendations and administer them at the correct rate.

THROMBOSIS

A thrombosis occurs when a blood clot on the cannula wall of the vein becomes detached and enters the pulmonary circulation. To prevent this from occurring we must:

- use the smallest size cannula to do the job required adequately
- avoid using veins in legs
- not flush the cannula if thromboembolism is suspected
- seek medical attention immediately.

Additional problems are what used to be called 'tissuing', but which should be called 'extravasation' or 'infiltration'.

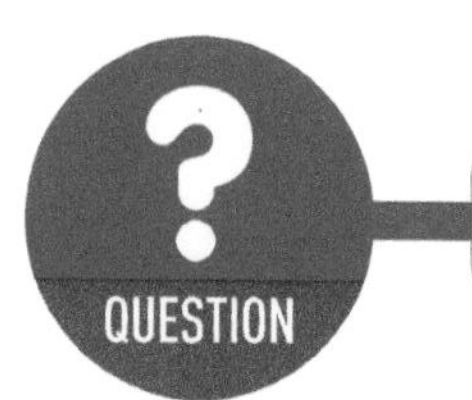

Question 12.2 What do the terms extravasation and infiltration mean?

Chapter 13 explains extravasation and infiltration in detail but, generally speaking, if large amount of fluids have infiltrated the surrounding tissues then swelling, pain and nerve damage may occur. Surgery may be required to drain the fluid.

REMOVING THE CANNULA

Cannulas are radio-opaque, meaning that they will show up under x-ray. This is important as we always need to check that we have retrieved the whole device on removal and that none of it has been left behind in the patient's body to migrate and cause damage.

Guidelines for the Cannulation Procedure

Equipment needed
Gloves and plastic apron
Appropriate size of cannula and a spare or two
Cleaning agent: a 70% isopropyl alcohol/2% chlorhexidine wipe (e.g. a Clinell swab); 2% chlorhexidine for adults, 0.05% for infants weighing <1.5 kg and 0.5% for those ≥ 1.5 kg. Use a 70% isopropyl alcohol wipe (e.g. Steret) or povidone iodine 10% if the patient is sensitive to chlorhexidine.
Cannula dressing
Long line attachment (primed with 0.9% sodium chloride) and 10 ml syringe with 0.9% sodium chloride
Tourniquet (preferably disposable)
Plastic sharps tray and sharps box
Alcohol gel

Procedure	
1	Explain the procedure to the patient and gain informed consent.
2	Ask the patient about their history of latex allergy prior to the procedure if there is no record of it.
3	Gather equipment together on a cleaned plastic tray with the sharps bin and take to the bedside.
4	Assist the patient into an appropriate position to allow access to the limb for cannulation.
5	Arrange the limb so that the patient is comfortable.
6	Apply the tourniquet, assess and select the appropriate vein and release the tourniquet.
7	Put on the plastic apron. Wash your hands using alcohol gel.
8	Open the outer plastic packaging and prepare the equipment.
9	Put on the gloves.
10	Clean the patient's skin and the selected vein thoroughly using selected skin cleaning fluid and allow to dry for 30 seconds. Do not repalpate the vein or touch the skin afterwards.
11	Reapply the tourniquet.
12	Remove the needle guard and inspect the device for any faults.
13	Anchor the vein by applying manual traction on the skin a few centimetres below the proposed site of insertion.

(Continued)

14	Ensure that the cannula is in the bevel-up position and insert it through the skin at the selected angle according to the depth of the vein. Forewarn the patient that the vein is about to be punctured by stating 'sharp scratch'.
15	Wait for the first flashback of blood in the flashback chamber of the stylet.
16	Level the device by decreasing the angle between the cannula and the skin and advance the cannula slightly to ensure entry into the lumen of the vein.
17	Withdraw the stylet slightly and a second flashback of blood will be seen along the shaft of the cannula.
18	Maintaining skin traction with the non-dominant hand and, using the dominant hand, slowly advance the cannula off the stylet and into the vein.
19	Release the vein.
20	Apply digital pressure to the vein above the cannula tip and remove the stylet immediately.
21	Dispose of the stylet into the sharps container. Attach the primed longline attachment and flush with 10 ml 0.9% sodium chloride using a push–pause technique.
22	Observe for signs of swelling or leakage and ask the patient if any pain or discomfort is felt (if appropriate). If any of these signs are evident, stop injecting the flush and remove the cannula.
23	Apply a fixation/dressing.
24	Discard the waste in the appropriate waste bins.
25	Remove your gloves and apron and wash your hands.
26	Document date, time, site of insertion, size of cannula and reason for insertion of the cannula in patients record (cannula care plan or equivalent; i.e. anaesthetic chart).

TEST YOUR KNOWLEDGE

1. Can a blood sample be obtained from a cannula?
2. What technique should be used to administer a flush?
3. What is the golden rule of cannula selection?
4. What is the approximate flow rate in litres/hour of a crystalloid fluid in a 22-gauge cannula?
5. What size syringe should we use to flush a cannula?

6. What does VIP stand for?
7. If an adult patient is sensitive to the cleaning fluid chlorhexidine, what can be used instead?
8. What is mechanical phlebitis?

KEY POINTS

- Selection of an appropriate device.
- Cannula selection.
- Approved sites and vein selection.
- Skin preparation and asepsis.
- Documentation and the VIP score.
- Problems associated with cannulation.

USEFUL WEB RESOURCES

B. Braun Medical Ltd. Peripheral IV Cannulation Training Programme. Quick reference guide: https://www.bbraun.co.uk/en/products-and-therapies/infusion-therapy/infusion-therapy-training.html

Geeky Medics. Intravenous cannulation (IV) OSCE guide: https://geekymedics.com/how-to-perform-cannulation-osce-guide

Chapter 13

INTRAVENOUS THERAPY

LEARNING OUTCOMES

By the end of this chapter you will have an understanding of the theory and practice of performing the clinical skill of intravenous (IV) therapy and knowledge of anaphylaxis.

The general pubic expects to receive the right drug at the right time under the right conditions and the government expects nothing less from NHS employees as part of clinical effectiveness.

It is now recognised practice that any qualified nursing, midwifery, radiography, registered operating department and anaesthetic practitioners and assistant practitioners who administer IV drugs must undertake a training programme, including an IV calculations test, and must be assessed as competent to carry out this skill.

In hospital environments, IV drugs are usually second-checked by a qualified member of staff. In community settings, this is not always possible and so extra care must be taken.

The above information is not intended to scare you, just to make you think very carefully about IV therapy and to highlight the fact that if you are not careful and vigilant then accidents and incidents can, and do, occur.

POSSIBLE COMPLICATIONS

The possible complications of IV therapy include:

- cannula occlusion/damage
- pain
- phlebitis
- embolism
- drug error
- needlestick injury
- speed shock/fluid overload/free flow

- extravasation
- infiltration
- haematoma.

We shall look at these complications individually.

Cannula Occlusion/Damage

We must never ignore a cannula occlusion as immediate action will be required.

A patient having IV drugs must have an access port in place, usually a peripheral venous catheter (PVC; see Chapter 12). The first thing we may notice with an occluded cannula is difficulty flushing the actual device. The patient may express pain at the cannula site, warranting an immediate resiting of a new cannula. If a patient is having IV fluids delivered via a pump then the pump alarms may be triggered. *Never ignore a pump alarm:* it will be sounding for a reason.

If the IV therapy was being administered without a pump – known as gravity feed – you may notice that the infusion has run very slowly or has even stopped at times.

When flushing a cannula you must use the push–pause technique with a 10-ml syringe or larger: nothing smaller than a 10-ml syringe should be used (see Chapter 12).

Never force a flush because it may cause a clot at the end of the PVC to be dislodged, which would lead to a thrombotic event.

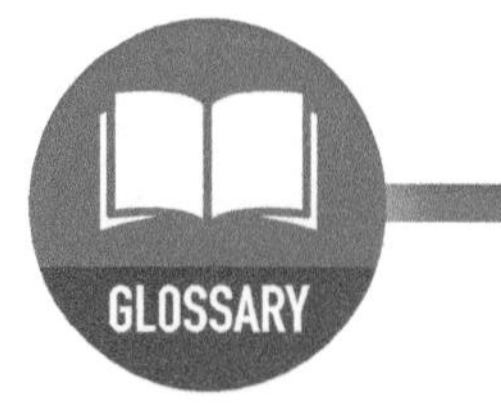

Thrombosis
The formation of a blood clot inside a blood vessel, obstructing the flow of blood through the circulatory system.

Pain

The cannula site should be inspected using the VIP score (meaning visual inspection of phlebitis; see Chapter 12). It should be remembered, however, that the patient's arm does not have to *look* painful to actually *be* painful.

Sometimes a cannula may have been sited in a poor position, such as over a joint, so that every time the joint is moved it causes pain. The cannula might also have become damaged.

A painful cannula site may also be due to the drug, perhaps if the wrong dilution has been used. Phenytoin has the same pH as bleach and can be very painful if a large cannula has been sited and has possibly migrated out of the vein. The drug then starts to cause extravasation, eating away at the surrounding tissues.

Above all, *listen to the patient.*

Phlebitis may also be a cause of pain; regular inspections should be made of the PVC device (see Chapter 12).

Embolism

There are three types of embolism:

- *Thrombus (blood clot):* this is usually treated with oral anticoagulants, in most cases with drugs such as warfarin. Daily or alternate-day international normalised ratios (INRs) should be obtained.
- *Air entering cardiovascular system*: this is why we exclude air from IV administration sets and syringes. It does not take very much air in the system to cause death; probably as little as 8–10 ml.
- *Mechanical:* this is caused by a broken piece of cannula, glass from an ampoule or rubber from an ampoule getting into the system. Studies have shown that 50% of glass ampoules have glass shards at the bottom following their being snapped open. This is why it is so important to change needles after the medication has been drawn up, before the injection.

You must also always check the cannula that you have removed. If you suspect that part of the tubing is missing, the patient will require an x-ray to locate the missing section, which will have to be removed surgically.

Drug Errors

More patients are requiring IV therapy today than ever before, so we need to be expert when administering medication via this route (as with all medications via all routes). However, up to 50% of all IV therapy drug administrations include a calculations error.

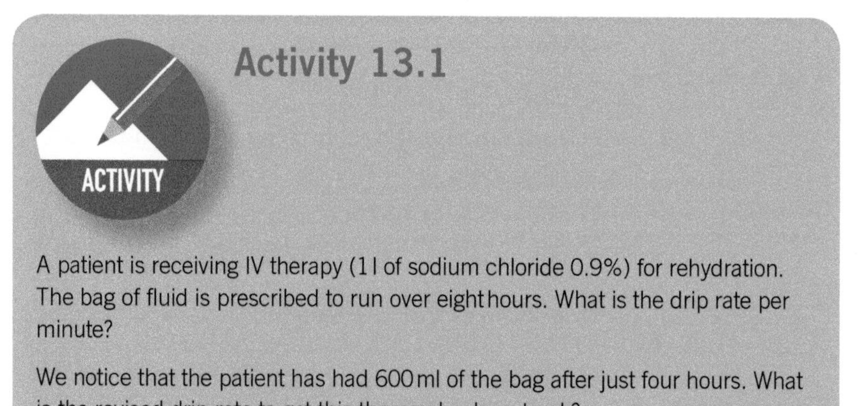

Activity 13.1

A patient is receiving IV therapy (1 l of sodium chloride 0.9%) for rehydration. The bag of fluid is prescribed to run over eight hours. What is the drip rate per minute?

We notice that the patient has had 600 ml of the bag after just four hours. What is the revised drip rate to get this therapy back on track?

What actions would you take?

For drug errors involving infusions, we would need to stop running the infusion immediately and inform senior staff, including the nurse in charge, medic and pharmacist. We should always inform our patients of drug-related mistakes and offer reassurance and undertake relevant observations. Documentation will need to be completed. Nurses must be honest, because the NHS is striving to learn from the mistakes in a 'non-blame culture' and to facilitate transparency so that patients to have renewed faith in their NHS.

Needlestick Injury

- Needlestick injuries are most often caused by re-sheathing needles: never re-sheath a needle.
- Data suggest that most injuries occur after the procedure, so put sharps straight into the sharps bin.
- Do not overfill sharps bins: they should only ever be three-quarters full or filled to the line markings before being sealed shut.
- Be careful when handling sharps: gloves will help to wipe off any of the patient's blood from a needle, minimising the amount of blood taken into your system.
- You should not use pulp trays, only clean rigid injection trays. Pulp trays are made from paper-mâché and when the trays are wet sharps can penetrate this material.
- Read your local sharps handling policy and know what to do if you are injured.

If you have a needlestick injury, *administer first aid:*

- encourage the wound to bleed by squeezing
- wash it thoroughly with running water
- cover the wound with waterproof dressing
- inform the nurse in charge and contact your local needlestick injury hotline and/or occupational health. Complete the necessary documentation.

Speed Shock/Fluid Overload/Free Flow

Speed shock is the rapid, uncontrolled administration of a drug, where symptoms occur as a result of the speed with which the medication is administered rather than the volume of drug or fluid. It can therefore occur even with small volumes. An example of this is a drug called furosemide which, if administered too fast, can cause tinnitus or permanent deafness. This drug has to be administered at a rate of 4 mg per minute.

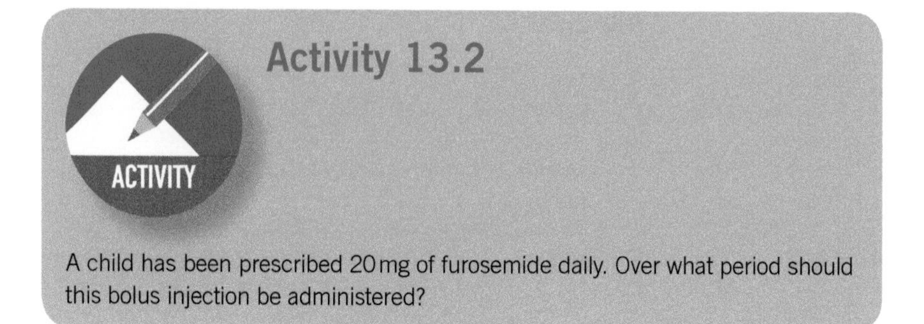

Activity 13.2

A child has been prescribed 20 mg of furosemide daily. Over what period should this bolus injection be administered?

When we add drugs to bags of fluids, we need to invert the bag several times to mix the mixture well. Otherwise, all the medication can fall to the bottom of the bag and be administered to the patient in far too concentrated a dose. (what if the drug was potassium? We could have a fatality on our hands.)

Fluid overload is literally when we overload our patients with fluids, such as the patient in Activity 13.1. This can be very dangerous in 'at-risk' patients, such as those with cardiac or renal disease, older patients and children.

Free flow is when the fluid we are administering is not regulated. Fluid overload can result.

The causes and complications of free flow are potentially very dangerous if patient is at risk (i.e. with cardiac failure). Avoid free flow by using a pump. If you are using a gravity feed, remember your drip rate formula. Observe the infusion frequently. Beware if the cannula is 'positional'; that is, improperly sited in the vein and prone to being dislodged. Confused patients may open a clamp or valve. Inform medical staff immediately if free flow has occurred. Perform accurate vital sign monitoring and document all incidents.

Extravasation

Extravasation is when a vesicant (blister-forming) substance eats away at the underlying tissue due to a cannula coming out of a vein (see also Chapter 12). It takes very little time for this to occur. Treatment is usually for adrenaline to be injected into the surrounding area and for saline or water flushes to dilute the drug in the patient's tissues. As much of the drug as possible may be drawn out using a needle and syringe. Ice is applied to the damaged area and analgesia prescribed to ease the patient's pain.

Many oncology drugs may cause extravasation, and children are particularly prone because they have smaller veins. Extravasation can therefore occur more frequently in these clinical areas.

Infiltration

Infiltration used to be referred to as 'tissuing'. Infiltration occurs when a cannula dislodges from the vein and the infused substance runs into the tissues. The arm can become oedematous (very swollen). Treatment is usually by raising the patient's arm so that the infusion may be absorbed slowly into the bodily tissues.

We know that infiltration can cause permanent nerve damage and a patient may require an escharotomy, surgery to 'spilt and drain' to remove this excess fluid. As little as 500 ml of fluid can cause permanent nerve damage.

Haematoma

Haematomas are caused by uncontrollable bleeding, usually creating a hard, discoloured, painful swelling under the skin.

Anaphylaxis

Another complication of administering IV medications, as with any medication, is the possibility of an anaphylactic event.

Allergic reactions (Figure 13.1) are caused by substances in the environment, known as allergens. Most commonly these are pollen from trees and grasses, frass from house dust mites, wasp and bee stings and certain foodstuffs, such as peanuts, milk and eggs. Asthma and skin disorders can also be allergy related.

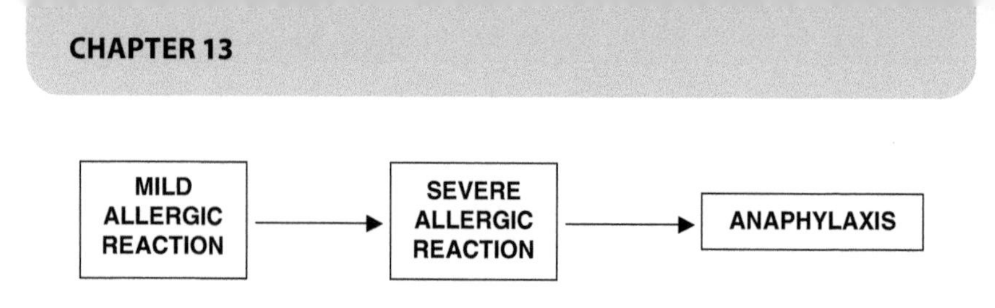

Figure 13.1 Types of allergic reaction.

One third of the UK population is now estimated to have an allergy, the most common one being caused by pollen from trees and grasses. Most allergic reactions can occur within minutes of exposure to the allergen, but some can present with a slower onset.

The UK Science and Technology Committee (a House of Lords committee) found that there has been a rapid growth in the number of people suffering from allergies, as a result of both genetic and environmental factors. The phenomenon has been described as an epidemic.

Milder allergic reactions, where there is no deterioration in cardiovascular or respiratory function, and which are not life-threatening, may not require any treatment.

Anaphylaxis is the most severe form of allergic reaction and is life-threatening because it does involve the airway, breathing and circulation, and can be triggered by a very broad range of agents. Each year, over 6000 people in England are admitted to hospital because of an allergy; one quarter of these people have anaphylaxis severe enough to be potentially life-threatening due to the involvement of the airways, causing breathing difficulties. People can die from anaphylaxis if treatment is not obtained quickly enough, as they go into anaphylactic shock (this is when the airway, breathing and circulation are involved). They may have presented initially with just a 'lump in the throat', tingling in the mouth or a rash. The UK Resuscitation Council reports an average of 20 deaths per year as a result of anaphylaxis, which they also state is likely to be a significant underestimation.

As a health carer you will be involved in drug administration, and we do not want those in our care to suffer an adverse reaction due to something that we have administered, be it food or medication. It is possible to aspirate the stomach contents by gastric lavage if a patient is given a drug to which they subsequently react or to remove medication that has been administered rectally or vaginally to minimise the exposure to the drug. When administering drugs by the IV route, we need to know about anaphylaxis and how to manage an adverse event. This is because IV drugs enter the body system quickly and there is no recall once the drug has been administered (although there is often an antidote).

WHAT IS ANAPHYLAXIS?

Anaphylaxis is likely when all of the following three criteria are met:

1 life-threatening and/or breathing and/or circulation problems
2 skin and/or mucosal changes
3 sudden onset and rapid progression of symptoms.

Anaphylaxis is defined as a severe, life-threatening and generalised or systemic hypersensitivity reaction.

In other words, anaphylaxis is an exaggerated response of a previously sensitised individual to a foreign antigenic material. The individual will therefore need to have had previous exposure to the substance (the antigen; see below for a discussion about allergens and antigens). However, there may be no knowledge by the individual of this previous exposure if the adverse effects were mild.

Phylaxis is a word seldom used in healthcare; it means 'protection' in Greek. So what do you think *anaphylaxis* means? It has the opposite meaning: 'without protection'.

WHAT IS AN ANAPHYLACTOID EVENT?

An anaphylactoid event occurs on first exposure to an antigen, so needs no specific antibody. If someone col-lapses, there is no need to stand over them and wonder

'Hmm! I wonder if this is an anaphylactic or an anaphylactoid event?' Both present with the same symptoms and require the same treatment. Both can be fatal. Subsequent events will be anaphylactic as, following the first event, antibodies will be made by the body. The antibodies will be triggered by exposure to the same antigen in the future.

This was misunderstood and for many years medics only gave the first IV antibiotic injections to patients, and nurses could only give the second or third doses. We now know that a reaction to an antibiotic is more likely to occur on the second dose onwards, when antibodies in the body recognise the antigen from last time and start an immune reaction.

Sometimes, individuals experience very mild symptoms on first exposure and do not recognise this as a reaction to a new drug or something they have just eaten.

WHAT'S THE DIFFERENCE BETWEEN AN ANTIBODY AND AN ANTIGEN?

An antibody is a protein produced by the immune system in response to the presence of an antigen, a protein that is in or on material that the body 'sees' as 'foreign'. An allergen is an antigen that causes an allergic reaction. The body attacks this 'enemy' material – the antigen – by producing antibodies. In an allergic reaction, this sets off a cascade of chemicals, such as histamines and cortisone, creating the symptoms of a severe reaction.

Such a reaction can affect the airway, breathing and circulation, resulting in the symptoms of *laryngeal oedema* (or swelling), *bronchospasm* and *hypotension*. As the throat is very vascular, swelling to this area may be the first sign that a problem is occurring. The patient may present with a rasping/husky voice.

Unfortunately, we can become allergic to anything at any time in our lifespan. Sometimes an anaphylactic reaction can present with symptoms and signs that are very similar to life-threatening asthma: this is most common in children.

There may also be confusion between an anaphylactic reaction and a panic attack. Victims of previous anaphylaxis can be prone to panic attacks if they think they have been re-exposed to the allergen that caused the previous problem. Other non-life-threatening conditions are:

- fainting (vasovagal episode)
- panic attack
- breath-holding in children
- idiopathic (non-allergic) urticaria or angioedema.

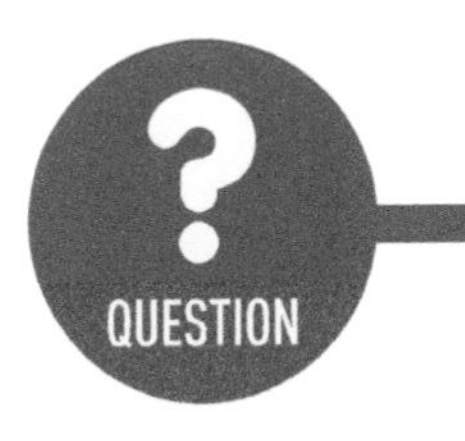

Question 13.1 Unravel the words to find the four most common trigger groups for an anaphylaxis event.

1 DOSOF
2 DETINCEJ MNOVE
3 GSRUD
4 TELAX

FOODS

In children, foods are the most common trigger for a severe allergic reaction, including:

- peanuts (about 1 in 200 people are allergic to them)
- tree nuts: walnuts, pecans, pistachios, cob nuts, cashews, almonds, etc.
- shellfish
- fish
- milk
- pulses: lentils
- sesame
- soy
- wheat
- eggs
- some fruit and vegetables.

Many foodstuffs, and other products, contain a problematic antigen that may not be obvious in the actual item. For instance, the main ingredient of some cardiac drugs is based on avocado, and people with dairy intolerance need to ensure that the outer casings of tablets do not contain milk proteins, which are commonly used in antibiotics.

Many breads or biscuits contain peanuts, or are produced in factories where peanut-based foods are also prepared, contaminating other non-peanut-based foodstuffs.
A shampoo often used to treat cradle cap contains peanuts: arachis oil. What a minefield! Thankfully, European regulations now require ingredients to be listed on food packaging.

INJECTED VENOM

Some of the known injected-venom triggers are:

- bees
- wasps
- yellow jackets
- hornets
- ants.

Why, do you think, is snake or spider venom not on the list? After all, many people like to keep exotic snakes and spiders from overseas. Well, I posed this question to a specialist and was informed that it is because it takes approximately five minutes to die of respiratory arrest following a potent spider or snake bite, which is not long enough for the cascade of chemicals to be released to cause an anaphylaxis event. In other words, the venom will kill you before the anaphylaxis will!

DRUGS

Medications are the most common trigger for anaphylaxis in adults. You may have seen television medical dramas in which someone undergoing an operation is asked by the anaesthetist, as they are slowly injecting the anaesthetic, 'any metallic taste in your mouth?' Or perhaps you have been asked this question while 'going under'. Do you know why? It is because a metallic taste in the mouth is often the first indication that someone is starting to react to a medication. Some other known drug triggers are:

- penicillin and cephalosporin antibiotics
- aspirin and non-steroidal anti-inflammatory drugs
- sulfa antibiotics
- allopurinol
- muscle relaxants
- vaccines
- radiocontrast media
- antihypertensives
- insulin
- blood products.

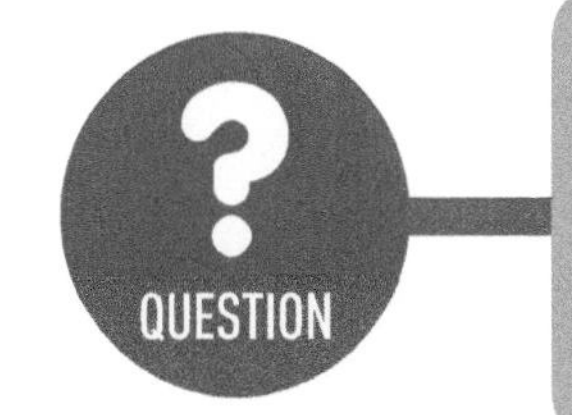

Question 13.2 Can you explain what the following drugs are for?

- Cephalosporin antibiotics
- Sulfa antibiotics
- Allopurinol

LATEX

We know that latex is all around us in nature. For instance, dandelion 'milk' contains latex. But the problematic substance is that from the rubber tree. In healthcare, exposure to this material commonly occurs via gloves. It has been estimated that less than 1% of the population is allergic to latex, but the problem is more prevalent among those working in healthcare and in the hairdressing industry. We also know that certain groups of individuals have an increased risk of sensitivity, such as people who have had multiple surgical procedures (due to latex proteins entering the body from the surgeon's gloves) and those who suffer from dermatitis, asthma or food allergies.

Patients who state on admission to hospital that they are allergic to certain fruits (the top three being bananas, avocado and kiwi fruits) must be treated as latex sensitive. Why? It is because these fruits contain similar protein chains to those found in latex. Therefore, we must not expose them to this protein. Many NHS trusts do not allow latex gloves in the workplace, except for 'high-risk' procedures and in surgery or during operations.

Foodstuffs and plants that contain similar protein chains to latex are:

- apples
- avocados
- bananas
- celery
- cherries
- chestnuts
- Ficus (trees of the fig family)
- figs
- grapes
- kiwi fruits
- mangoes
- melons
- passion fruit
- peaches
- pears
- pistachios
- potatoes
- ragweed
- strawberries
- tomatoes.

ROUTES

Anaphylaxis does not only occur with medication being administered via the IV route, although this is a very quick mode of entry. Any of the bodily routes can cause a reaction to occur, because the allergen has entered the body, such as:

- orally
- rectally
- vaginally
- inhaled
- subcutaneously
- intravenously
- topically.

WHAT ARE THE SIGNS AND SYMPTOMS OF ANAPHYLAXIS?

Although we have discussed how a true anaphylactic event has airway, breathing and circulatory involvement, anaphylaxis can be broken up into five areas of response:

1. cutaneous
2. respiratory
3. central nervous system
4. gastrointestinal
5. cardiovascular.

Cutaneous

Cutaneous pertains to the skin. An individual may have a reaction to something that causes skin involvement; this may or may not go on to cause an anaphylactic reaction, and so it should be treated promptly. Cutaneous involvement may present as:

- swelling (angio-oedema)
- urticaria (hives)
- redness (erythema)
- itching (pruritus)
- sweating.

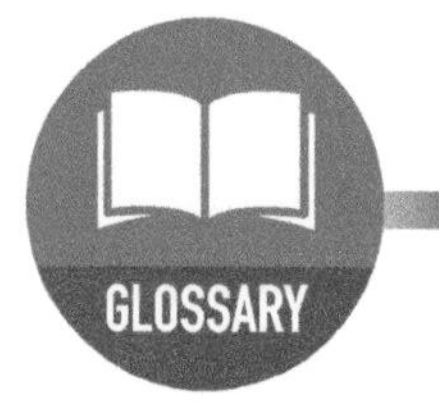

Rhinitis

Inflammation of the membranes lining the nose, causing extreme running of secretions or sometimes blockage. Antihistamines may relieve the symptoms.

Stridor

High-pitched noise heard on inspiration, caused by upper airway obstruction. This is a medical emergency.

Angio-oedema may cause occlusion of the airway. The urticaria can be painful as well as unsightly, as may erythema. Pruritus may present as a maddening itch, which can occur when an individual is having a reaction to penicillin. Chlorphenamine maleate, more commonly known by its trade name Piriton®, may be prescribed in this case to relieve the irritation.

Reassuringly, most patients who have skin changes caused by allergy do not go on to develop an anaphylactic reaction.

Respiratory

Respiratory involvement may start off as a 'lump in the throat'. This is due to laryngeal oedema as the airways are starting to close over. Other respiratory involvement may include:

- wheezing
- dyspnoea, with increased respiratory rate
- rhinitis
- laryngeal obstruction leading to stridor
- hypoxia
- respiratory arrest.

Any difficulty breathing is life-threatening. Oxygen should be administered and the airway cleared, with a laryngeal adjunct, if necessary. But the most important thing is to *call for help*.

Central Nervous System

A patient may first experience a feeling of faintness and/or dizziness due to a lowering of blood pressure: hypotension. Other signs may be:

- confusion (due to hypoxia)
- feeling of impending doom
- apprehension/anxiety
- metallic taste in the mouth
- altered level of consciousness.

Initially, it may be difficult to distinguish whether a patient is confused by being in hospital and losing their bearings or whether the confusion is the start of a reaction to a drug that has not long been administered, causing decreased oxygen brain perfusion. The 'feeling of impending doom' is a strange one, as this indicates central nervous system involvement. I have only ever seen this once in my nursing career, whereby a patient asked me tell his wife that she was 'a wonderful woman' before he collapsed!

Gastrointestinal

Depending on an individual's trigger, injected drugs can have a quicker reaction than injected venom (stings), which in turn have a quicker reaction than orally ingested triggers. Gastrointestinal symptoms may not be immediately life-threatening (but in very small children and the elderly this *will* be more critical).

Cardiovascular

Remember that true anaphylaxis involves the airway, breathing and circulation. Initially, a patient may present with signs of shock, becoming pale and clammy, and feeling faint and dizzy. Other signs of cardiovascular symptoms are:

- hypotension
- tachycardia
- cardiac arrhythmias
- cardiac arrest.

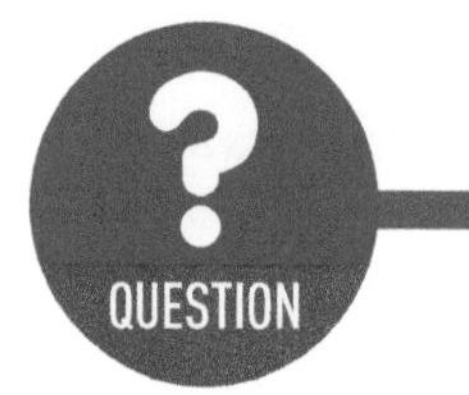

Question 13.3 Would you sit someone up whom you suspected of having an anaphylaxis event?

MANAGEMENT

Prevention is always better than cure, so the best prevention is not to expose our patients to a known allergen!

It is important that we know our patients well, by making a good assessment on admission, if in hospital, and checking our patient's history of adverse reactions before prescribing or administering any medication. After any new treatment, patients should always remain in the location for at least 10 minutes so that we can observe for any adverse reactions. Medical treatment can be given immediately in this situation, if required. How many of you have been given a vaccine, perhaps for influenza or when going on holiday. Hopefully you were asked to sit down and observed for this amount of time. Anyone experiencing a reaction should be laid flat, with feet raised, given oxygen (if available) and given the first line of treatment: adrenaline. As with any emergency situation, the ABCDE assessment will be performed:

A Airway
B Breathing
C Circulation
D Disability
E Exposure.

Patients could have either an A, B, or C problem or any combination. Table 13.1 shows how the ABCDE assessment relates to an anaphylactic event.

It is important to remember that a patient should receive immediate medical treatment when experiencing symptoms indicative of anaphylaxis. The flowchart in Figure 9.2 shows healthcare management of an anaphylactic event.

Table 13.1 ABCDE assessment and anaphylaxis.

Assessment	Symptoms
A	Airway swelling, e.g. throat and tongue swelling (pharyngeal/laryngeal oedema). The patient has difficulty breathing and swallowing and feels that the throat is closing up.
B	See Respiratory section under 'What are the signs and symptoms of anaphylaxis?'
C	See Cardiovascular section under 'What are the signs and symptoms of anaphylaxis?'
D	Airway, breathing and circulation problems also alter the patient's neurological status due to decreased brain perfusion. The patient's blood glucose should be obtained to rule out hypoglycaemia and the prescription chart should also be checked. See the section of this chapter on the central nervous system under 'What are the signs and symptoms of anaphylaxis?'
E	Fully expose the body and examine the patient thoroughly. Remember to minimise heat loss and to maintain the patient's dignity. Remember to call for help. See the cutaneous section of this chapter under 'What are the signs and symptoms of anaphylaxis?'

ADRENALINE

In the hospital environment, adrenaline (epinephrine) is located on the resuscitation trolley in the 'first-line' emergency drug box. Nurses working in the community should have easy access to their supplies of adrenaline.

Adrenaline for anaphylaxis is expressed as 1 : 1000, which means that there is 1 mg of the drug in every 1 ml of fluid (1 g in 1000 ml). In an emergency, nurses can administer 0.5 ml (0.5 mg or 500 μg) intramuscularly (IM), usually in the more assessable mid outer thigh: the vastus lateralis muscle. As time is of the essence, it may not be appropriate to remove outer clothes, such as tights and/or trousers.

Five minutes later, a second injection of 0.5 ml/0.5 mg can be given. Some adrenaline comes ready prepared in the syringe; in some areas you may have to draw it up yourself. It is important not to get confused with adrenaline administered for cardiopulmonary resuscitation: this is expressed as 1:10 000, which means 1 mg in every 10 ml. Although this is a larger volume (1 g in 10000 ml) it is more potent as it is given intravenously.

In many clinical areas, staff can only administer adrenaline when key factors are in place. They must follow Resuscitation Council (UK) requirements, have attended an IV study day, be up to date with their basic life support training, have attended anaphylaxis training and been assessed as competent. Figure 13.2 shows the Resuscitation Council (UK)'s algorithm for the treatment of an anaphylactic event.

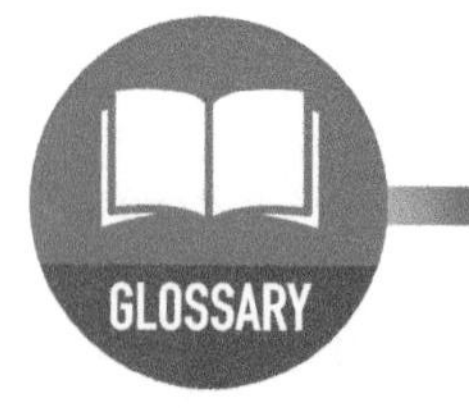

Phaeochromocytoma

A tumour of the adrenal glands. Symptoms may include headache, sweating, hypertension and palpitations.

How Does Adrenaline Work?

Now for the scientific bit! During anaphylaxis, the blood vessels leak, bronchial tissues swell, and the blood pressure drops, causing the choking and collapse.

Adrenaline acts quickly to:

- constrict the blood vessels
- relax the smooth muscles in the lungs to improve breathing
- stimulate the heart's contractility
- help to stop swelling around the face and lips (the angio-oedema).

AFTERCARE

After an episode of anaphylaxis, the patient will need reassurance, rest and continued observation. They will also need to receive health education about why this episode happened and be advised to avoid the trigger, if possible, in the future. Many patients like to carry a patient information in the form of a medical alert bracelet in case they are unable to communicate verbally at the time of an attack.

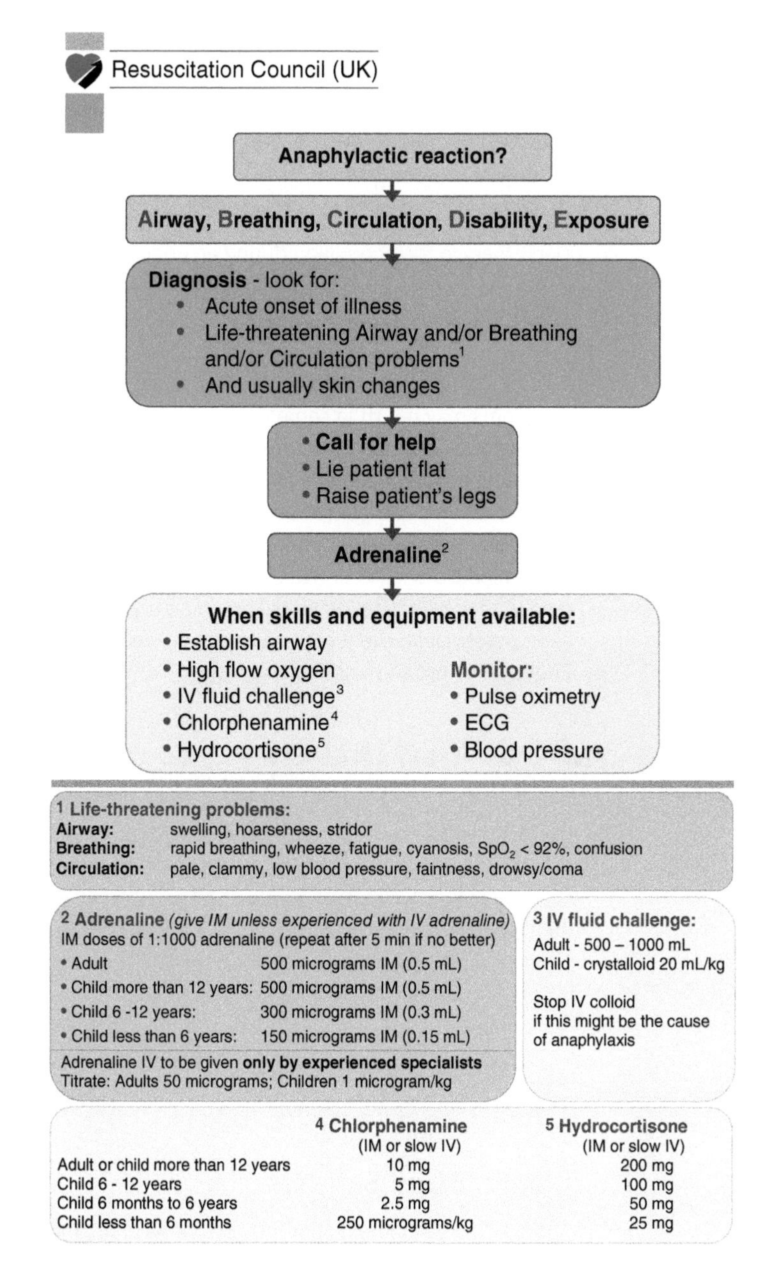

Figure 13.2 Treatment for an anaphylactic event. Source: Permission to reproduce this image is granted by the Resuscitation Council (UK).

Healthcare professionals may also complete a yellow card, found in the British National Formulary (BNF; https://bnf.nice.org.uk), to alert the Department of Health that a particular drug has caused an adverse reaction.

Patients can also carry a Lifeline card (https://www.lifelinehelpline.info/page/lifeline-campaign.html), again to alert others to their condition during an anaphylactic event.

BIPHASIC RESPONSE

A biphasic response is known as a 'rebound', whereby the symptoms may return in some people after the initial episode and treatment. Recurrence can be 8–12 hours after the first attack, and patients should always be informed of this so that they can plan to be not alone. Further doses of adrenaline may be required. It is always good practice to give patients a booklet or leaflet with information for them to read in their own time, as verbal information given during their anaphylactic event may be forgotten. Remember, English may not be their first language.

DOCUMENTATION

If the incident occurred in a hospital, a description of the reaction, with circumstances, timings, treatments and investigations must be documented. If the incident occurred when a blood product was being administered then paperwork relating to this will need to be completed. Any suspected substance/drug/allergen should be kept while the investigation is being completed.

INVESTIGATIONS OF ANAPHYLAXIS

Clotted Blood Samples

The specific test to help confirm a diagnosis of an anaphylactic reaction is measurement of mast cell tryptase. This is taken in a blood sample obtained via venepuncture. Tryptase levels are useful in the follow-up of suspected anaphylactic reactions, not in the initial recognition and treatment. The half-life of mast cell tryptase is short (approximately two hours) and concentrations may be back to normal levels within six to eight hours, so the timing of any blood samples is very important.

Urine

Urine samples may also be collected immediately after the reaction and then again two to four hours after the incident. This is obtained to measure methylhistamine. Methylhistamine is what histamine turns into when your body inactivates it.

Immunology Therapy

Immunology therapy is when small doses of antigen are injected into patients to decrease reactions to subsequent exposures. These patients are obviously closely watched for any reactions and all tests are conducted over very strict laboratory conditions. There has been some degree of success with children exposed to peanuts.

Skin Tests

Skin tests are the only way we have to tell us what the person had a reaction too. The blood and urine sample tests for mast cell tryptase and methylhistamine just tell us that a person has had a reaction. Very often patients have to pay privately for these tests.

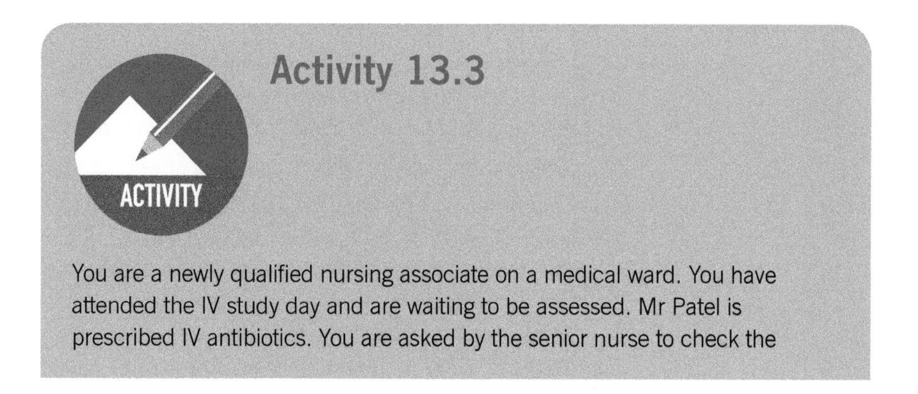

Activity 13.3

You are a newly qualified nursing associate on a medical ward. You have attended the IV study day and are waiting to be assessed. Mr Patel is prescribed IV antibiotics. You are asked by the senior nurse to check the antibiotics with him. You notice that he does not wash his hands before drawing up the drugs, but do not feel that you can challenge him. You subsequently notice that he does not wear gloves during the preparation of the antibiotics. After drawing up the antibiotics, you check them and all seems fine. You check the patient against the drug chart and all is correct. The senior nurse sits on the edge of the bed and places the pulp tray on the bed next to him. He is about to start giving the antibiotics when the ward clerk asks him to take a phone call. As he gets up, he leaves the tray and contents on the bed. He returns to the patient and, without inspecting the cannula, administers the antibiotics. In the clinical room, he empties the contents of the tray into the sharps bin, one syringe and needle does not quite go all the way in, so he 'pushes' it in, receiving a needle stick injury. You notice that the bin is very full. What mistakes have been made?

PROCEDURE FOR THE ADMINISTRATION OF IV FLUIDS VIA GRAVITY

1. Collect all the necessary equipment.
2. Wash your hands.
3. Gloves must be worn if giving antibiotic therapy (sterile gloves are not required). Two checkers are required for IV therapy.
4. Apply aseptic principles.
5. Check that you are with the correct patient and gain consent.
6. Inspect the fluid bag to be certain that it contains the correct fluid, the fluid is clear (if the medication should be), the bag is not leaking and the bag has not expired.
7. Sterile packaging must not be damaged or wet.
8. Ensure that you have the correct giving set for the fluid to be administered, as different sets are required for blood and blood products and for electronic devices. These sets are either microdrip sets, which deliver 60 drops per ml into the drip chamber, or macrodrip sets, which deliver 15–20 drops per ml into the drip chamber.

9 Open the packaging and uncoil the tubing: do not let the ends of the tubing become contaminated. Close the flow regulator (roll the wheel away from the end to which you will attach the fluid bag).

10 Remove the protective covering from the port of the fluid bag and the protective covering from the spike of the administration set.

11 Insert the spike of the administration set into the port of the fluid bag with a quick twist. Do this carefully. Be especially careful not to puncture yourself! Insert this spike fully into the infusion bag, as this is an infection risk.

12 Hold the fluid bag higher than the drip chamber of the administration set. Squeeze the drip chamber once or twice to start the flow. Fill the drip chamber to one-third full. If you overfill the chamber, lower the bag below the level of the drip chamber and squeeze some fluid back into the fluid bag.

13 Open the flow regulator and allow the fluid to flush all the air from the tubing. Let it run into the giving set's empty packaging or container.
You may need to loosen or remove the cap at the end of the tubing to get the fluid to flow to the end of the tubing (but this should not be necessary), taking care not to let the tip of the administration set become contaminated.

14 The primed giving set is now ready to be connected to an electronic device or the rate can be determined by gravity flow together with the flow clamp.

15 Connect the end of the tubing to the patient: the IV cannula must be of an appropriate size for the intended use and cleaned before the administration set line end is attached, to minimise infection risk.

16 Document the procedure and initiate a fluid chart document.

TEST YOUR KNOWLEDGE

Questions 1 and 2 are are scenario exercises. You may wish to see if you can borrow copy of the British National Formulary (BNF) for this exercise or just have a go at answering as much as you can.

1 Mrs Jones is admitted to hospital with a systemic bacterial infection, thought to be respiratory in origin. She has been prescribed metronidazole 500 mg QDS (four times a day) and cefuroxime 750 mg QDS. You are a third-year student nurse on your last placement. The nurse you are working with is a registered general nurse (RGN) and is very experienced at administering IV medication.

The RGN mixes the two antibiotics together, ready for the midnight dose. You are asked to check the medication. You assume that the two antibiotics can be mixed, as this nurse is very experienced. You check the medication and all seems fine, all is in date and prescribed for the right patient. You go through the checks:

- right medicine
- right dose
- right route
- right patient
- right time.

The RGN checks the patient's identity bands to check that this is the correct patient and administers the medication without any problems and disposes of the sharps correctly. The drug chart is signed appropriately.

At 02:30 the patient complains of feeling nauseous and has developed diarrhoea. She states she feels very unwell. The clinical site manager is paged and shortly arrives on the ward. The manager looks at the drug chart and at once notices the mistake.

What mistakes have been made?

2. You are a community nurse. When you are attending to Mrs Halfpenny, you notice that the cannulation site is red and the redness is tracking up her arm. When you question her, you are told that the redness has developed 24 hours ago. The nurse who administered the previous dose told her that it was expected of an IV antibiotic.
3. What do you think is happening in this scenario?
4. What is the main generating trigger for an anaphylactic event in children?
5. What is the main generating trigger for an anaphylactic event in adults?
6. What is angio-oedema?
7. Name some of the known food triggers for anaphylaxis.

KEY POINTS

- Possible complications of IV therapy.
- Procedure for the administration of IV fluids via the gravity procedure.
- Anaphylaxis.

USEFUL WEB RESOURCES

Anaphylaxis Campaign: www.anaphylaxis.org.uk
British National Formulary: https://bnf.nice.org.uk
Epipen®: www.epipen.com
Lifeline campaign: https://www.lifelinehelpline.info/page/lifeline-campaign.html
Resuscitation Council (UK): www.resus.org.uk
IB Boost UK. What is IV therapy?: https://ivboost.uk/about/what-is-iv-therapy-definition-benefits-types

Chapter 14

BLOOD TRANSFUSION

LEARNING OUTCOMES

By the end of this chapter you will have an understanding of the theory and practice of performing the clinical skill of administering a blood transfusion or blood products.

Blood transfusion is one of the clinical skills student nurses can take part in, but only in *part* of the process. This is also considered a mandatory training session, which you will probably receive in your induction to an NHS trust, and you will be expected to update your competency assessments every two years, but as with all clinical skills, you will need to check this with your own employer's policies and procedures.

Before we begin, let's look at the blood groups.

BLOOD GROUPS

The main blood groups are: O, A, B and AB. There is also an antibody known as D Rhesus antigen or Rh D. If this antigen is present, your blood group is known as *positive*. If this antigen is not present, your blood group is known as *negative*. The blood groups now look like Table 14.1.

Did you know, there are also rare blood groups, such as C, E, K, Fy, JK and S?

The O blood group is often referred to as the universal donor, as we can all receive blood from this group (Table 14.2).

Table 14.1 Blood groups.

O positive	**O negative**
A positive	**A negative**
B positive	**B negative**
AB positive	**AB negative**

Table 14.2 Blood group donors.

Blood group	Blood groups that can be a donor
O	O only
A	A and O
B	B and O
AB	A, B and O

To donate blood in the UK you need to be:

- fit and healthy
- weigh between 7 stone 12 lbs and 25 stone (50–158 kg)
- aged between 17 and 66 years (or 70 if you have given blood before)
- over 70 years and have given a full blood donation in the past two years.

Men can give blood every 12 weeks, while women can give blood every 16 weeks.

Each donation is for approximately 470 ml and just one donation can save up to three people's lives. Four percent of the population donate their blood, but 98% of us state that 'everyone should donate'!

DID YOU KNOW?

Whatever you do in life, always give 100%. Unless you give blood!

Strict regulations are in place concerning blood matters, from the Department of Health. Part of this concerns training: those who 'manufacture', collect, transport and store the blood, and those who deliver the products (i.e. drivers) must receive training.

The Serious Hazards of Transfusion (SHOT) organisation oversees the practice of blood transfusion and collects data across the UK on all transfusion reactions, adverse events or 'near-miss' events, from which we can learn from our mistakes. The SHOT report from 2020 showed us that there were 2.1 million blood components issued by the four blood services in 2020 (Table 14.3). The four blood services in the UK are:

1. NHS Blood and Transport
2. Northern Ireland
3. Scottish National Blood Transfusion Service
4. Welsh Blood Services.

DID YOU KNOW?

You may be wondering what methylene blue fresh frozen plasma (FFP) is. Babies' blood products are 'cleaned' and filtered further with a substance called methylene blue, which makes their urine blue and sometimes gives their skin a blue tinge (no wonder their families call them Smurf babies!). The methylene blue inactivates viruses, such as HIV and hepatitis C, and reduces the already small chance of viral transmission even further.

BLOOD PRODUCTS

As you can see from Table 14.3, it is not just whole blood that is transfused. Have you ever wondered what the different products are and what they are used to treat? Then wonder no more, as Table 14.4 looks at the products, a description of the products and what they are used for.

TRANSFUSION ERRORS

- The risk of serious harm related to transfusion in the UK is 1 in 15 142 components issued.
- The risk of death related to transfusion in the UK is 1 in 53 193 components issued (SHOT, 2021).

These errors can be broken down into three categories: preventable errors, possibly preventable errors and not preventable errors (Table 14.5).

Table 14.3 Total issues of blood components from the blood services of the UK, 2020.

	Red cells	Platelets	FFP	SD-FFP	MB-FFP	Cryo	Total
NHS Blood and Transport	1 286 287	230 792	145 101	61 069	5705	36.414	1 765 368
Northern Ireland	36 821	7280	2822	630	390	794	48 737
Scottish National Blood Transfusion	126 093	21 653	13 196	3040	374	2651	167 007
Welsh Blood Services	74 494	9046	6758	2730	—	377	93 405
Total	1 523 695	268 771	167 877	67 489	6489	40 236	2 074 517

FFP, fresh frozen plasma; SD, solvent detergent treated; MB, methylene-blue treated; Cryo, cryoprecipitate.
Source: SHOT (2021).

Table 14.4 Blood and blood products used in transfusion.

Product	Description	Indication for use
Red cells in additive solutions (saline, adenine, glucose and mannitol = SAGE)	Red cells with plasma removed and 100 ml additive used as replacement	Correction of anaemia
Washed red blood cells	Leuco-depleted (leucocytes, white blood cells, have been removed)	Correction of anaemia where patient may react to plasma components
Frozen red blood cells	Red cells of very rare phenotype; leuco-depleted	Used to treat patients with very rare antibody
White blood cells (granulocytes removed)	Mainly granulocytes removed from fresh blood (granulocytes are the most common type of white blood cell)	Used to treat patients with life-threatening granulocytopenia
Platelets	Platelets in 200–300 ml plasma	Used to treat thrombocytopenia (to prevent bleeding or treat bleeding)
FFP	Plasma separated from whole blood and treated with sodium citrate to prevent clotting	Used to treat multifactor deficiencies associated with severe bleeding
Albumin 4.5%	Solution of albumin from pooled plasma in a 0.9% sodium chloride solution	Used to treat hypovolaemic shock or hypoproteinaemia due to burns, trauma, surgery or infection
Albumin 20%	Heat-treated, aqueous, chemically processed fraction of pooled plasma	(As above indication for albumin 4.5%) to maintain appropriate electrolyte balance
Cryoprecipitate	Cold-insoluble portion of plasma recovered from FFP; rich in clotting factors; factor VIII, factor XIII, Von Willebrand factor and fibrinogen	Used to treat hypofibrinogenaemia (for those whose blood does not clot properly to prevent or control bleeding)
Solvent-treated FFP	Solvent detergent process inactivates bacteria and most encapsulated viruses	Used for treating thrombotic thrombocytopenic purpura

FFP, fresh frozen plasma.

Table 14.5 Transfusion errors.

Abbreviation	Error	Incidence (n)
Preventable		$N = 3214$
NM	Near miss	1130
Anti-D	Anti-D immunoglobulin errors	400
IBCT	Incorrect blood component transfused	323
HSE	Handling and storage errors	278
RBRP	Right blood, right patient	207
ADU	Delayed transfusion	133
ADU	Avoidable transfusion	110
ADU	Over or under transfusion	25
ADU	Prothrombin complex concentrates	17
Possibly preventable		
TACO	Transfusion-associated circulatory overload	149
HTR	Haemolytic transfusion reactions	46
TTI	Transfusion-transmitted infection	1
Not preventable		
FAHR	Febrile, allergic and hypotensive reactions	321
TAD	Transfusion-associated dyspnoea	37
CS	Cell salvage	23
UCT	Uncommon complications of transfusion	12
TRALI	Transfusion related acute lung injury	2
PTP	Post transfusion purpura	<3214 = 0
TAG vs HD	Transfusion-associated graft-vs-host disease	<3214 = 0

Source: Serious Hazards of Transfusion (SHOT) Report 2020.

DID YOU KNOW?

Did you notice that transfusion related acute lung injury (TRALI) is stated as 2, but this is actually 2 × 3214 = 6428 in numbers. As both Post transfusion purpura and Transfusion-associated graft-vs-host disease numbers are below the *n* number (3214), they are recorded as zero.

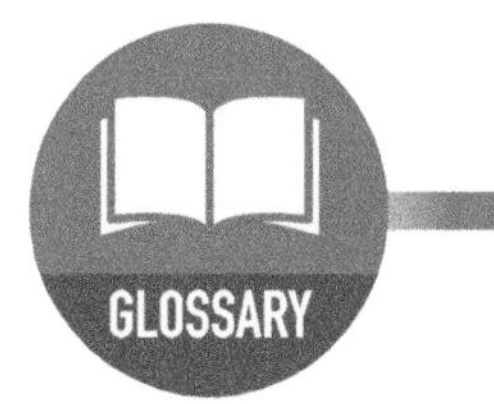

Post transfusion purpura
Haemorrhages in the skin and mucous membranes that result in the appearance of purple spots or patches.

It is therefore vital that vigilance is required when administering blood products to our patients, to minimise mistakes. This begins with consent and informing patients so that they can make an informed choice. Today, much of the transfusion process is automated.

CONSENT AND INFORMATION LEAFLETS

Before a patient receives a blood transfusion or a blood product, consent must be documented in their notes and a consent form signed. Patients should at this stage have their hospital identification bands in place (usually around their wrists). Figure 14.1 shows what the transfusion record looks like. It is pink in colour. Consent can only be obtained by a doctor or specialist nurse. The patient must also be given a patient information leaflet. As blood is such a precious commodity, the rationale for the patient receiving this 'tissue transplant' must also be written in their notes.

A preassessment clinic might wish a patient to increase the iron in their diet before being admitted for surgery, to increase their haemoglobin levels.

There are also very strict protocols for the use of blood by surgeons: for example, a surgeon can only order two units of blood for hip-replacement surgery, two units of blood for craniotomy neurosurgery, and so on.

It must be remembered that these leaflets come in other languages, as English may not be a patient's first language. The information leaflets are national, but some NHS trusts may produce their own patient information leaflets.

North Bristol NHS
NHS Trust

BLOOD TRANSFUSION RECORD

It is Trust policy to complete as a minimum:
Section 1: Indication for Transfusion Section 3: Agreement to Transfusion Section 4: Prescription
Section 5: Blood Collection Record of Administration: to record date, time & staff signatures

Hospital..	Affix patient addressograph here or complete below:
Ward/Dept...	**Surname:** ....
Directorate...	**First Name(s):** ....
Consultant...	**Hospital No:** .... **DOB** ....

1. **Indication for Transfusion**

An Hb threshold of **7g/dl** in otherwise fit patients (8g/dl in older patients and those with known / likely cardiovascular disease) is recommended unless symptomatic or active bleeding.
Transfusion to an Hb above 10g/dl is very rarely indicated unless patient is red cell dependent or a neonate.

Symptoms / signs ....

Diagnosis causing low Hb / anaemia / bleeding...

2. **Relevant Medical History** Special considerations.................................

Pre-transfusion Haemoglobin ....g/dl Blood group ....

Previous transfusion / blood product Yes / No Previous reaction:Yes / No When: ....

If yes, what and when? ....

3. **Agreement to Transfusion**

This patient has verbally agreed to a blood transfusion and has received relevant information leaflets or

this patient has not provided consent because...

Date .... Staff signature.................................. Print name ....

4. **Prescription**

Sections 1, 2 and 3 should be completed with prescription, except when 2 & 3 can be done pre-operation
N.B During surgery, prescription on an anaesthetic record is an acceptable alternative

Product & Amount	Date for infusion	Special requirements	Rate	Dr name, sign, date & time

5. **Blood Collection** (Take blood transfusion record to fridge) *(Requestor & Receiver please sign, and record date & time)*

		Unit 1	Unit 2	Unit 3	Unit 4	Unit 5	Unit 6
Requestor: check patient ID at bedside, patient ID confirmed with collector	Sign:	....	....	....	....	....	....
	Date	....	....	....	....	....	....
	Time	....	....	....	....	....	....
Receiver: take receipt of blood	Sign:	....	....	....	....	....	....
	Date	....	....	....	....	....	....
	Time	....	....	....	....	....	....

Page 1 of 2 Blood Transfusion Record February 2008 RVJ0694 (LGD)

Figure 14.1 Blood transfusion record. Source: Permission to reproduce this image is granted by North Bristol NHS Trust and University Hospitals Bristol NHS Foundation Trust.

It should also be remembered that not all patients will be hospital inpatients, and those who are not will require an information sheet to take home after their daycase transfusion.

Other information leaflets concern children and FFP and guides for parents of children or babies who are receiving blood products.

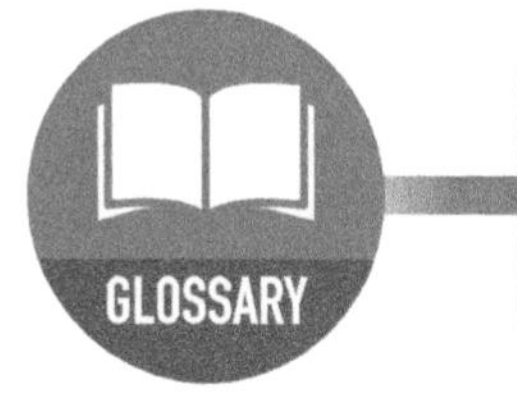

Fresh frozen plasma

The liquid component of human blood that has been frozen for preservation. It is thawed before administration.

BLOOD TRANSFUSION REQUESTS

Doctors or specialist nurses request blood after consent has been obtained on a blood transfusion request form. There may be specialist requirements, such as for washed cells, cytomegalovirus (CMV) or irradiated blood.

ACTIVITY

Activity 14.1

Have you ever heard of these blood products? What do you think they mean?

- Washed cells
- CMV
- Irradiated blood

The Blood Transfusion Request Form

The blood transfusion request form must be signed by a doctor or specialist nurse and must contain certain pieces of information: the patient's first name, surname, date of birth and hospital number. Special care must be taken with admissions to hospital with no hospital number, making a patient unable to give identification details.

SAMPLE COLLECTION

A blood sample must be collected by venepuncture to perform a crossmatch to check the patient's blood group. Venepuncture (see Chapter 11) can be performed by a doctor, phlebotomist or other staff trained in venepuncture, namely:

- a registered nurse
- a nursing associate
- a registered midwife
- an assistant practitioner
- a healthcare assistant.

Samples for crossmatching are obtained in a blood transfusion tube, known as an EDTA (ethylenediamine tetra-acetic acid) tube. The tubes usually have a red top to identify them as such. Tubes should be labelled at the bedside and gently inverted to mix the blood with the anticoagulant in the tube. Blood for crossmatching is sent to the same place that all samples are sent: the pathology laboratory.

COLLECTING BLOOD THAT HAS BEEN REQUESTED

Pre-collection Procedure

Before collecting blood, and after confirming that the blood is ready for collection, a cannula must be inserted or checked to establish patency. Check that you have any equipment needed, such as a filtered blood administration set, volumetric pump or blood warmer, if required. Baseline observations must also now be taken:

- temperature
- pulse
- blood pressure
- respiratory rate.

Now go back to the blood transfusion record and you will see that the requestor needs to sign, at the bottom of the document, that they have sent an individual to collect the blood. The requestor must check that the person they are sending has received blood transfusion training and is up to date with their competency. The person collecting the blood must take this record sheet with them to collect the blood.

Collection Procedure

As stated, collection requires appropriately trained staff.

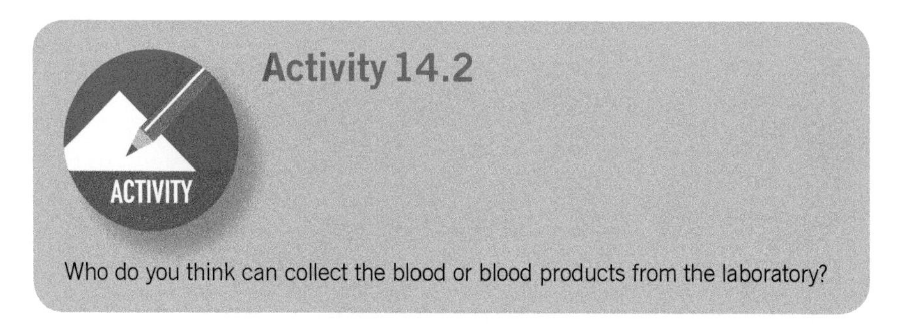

Activity 14.2

Who do you think can collect the blood or blood products from the laboratory?

Before you open the fridge containing the units of blood, you need to check the information you have on the blood transfusion record and the blood register, checking that all the details correspond:

- first name
- surname
- date of birth
- hospital number.

As previously stated, this process may be automated, using barcodes. Any discrepancies should be reported immediately. Then take the blood, which should have compatibility form attached (first unit only), much like a luggage label.

Note: only take *one bag of blood,* even if the patient has been prescribed more than one unit.

Operating theatres tend to use specialist cool boxes, which can keep the units cold for up to six hours. Only theatres can take more than one unit at a time, using these boxes, as they need to have the blood available during surgical procedures.

Check the blood for any signs of leaks or clots.

Check all the details on the compatibility label and the bag of blood and then sign the bag out in the blood register, stating the time that the blood was removed from the fridge. The blood should be transported to the clinical area in a specialised transit bag or covered so that it is not on full view to other patients and visitors while being transported.

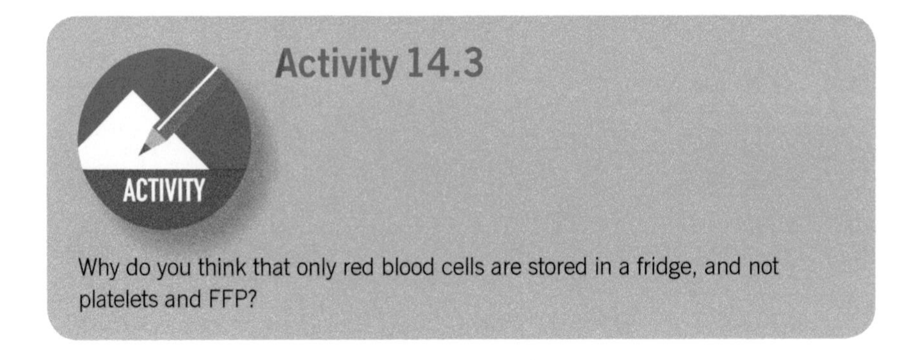

Activity 14.3

Why do you think that only red blood cells are stored in a fridge, and not platelets and FFP?

Receipt of Blood

Take the blood back to the clinical area and hand it to the requestor. The person taking receipt of the unit should check the patient's details on the compatibility label, compatibility report form and the blood transfusion record. They should then sign the blood transfusion record and record the date and time.

COLD-CHAIN REQUIREMENTS

The cold chain relates to the storage and temperature of blood and blood products, and is strictly monitored.

- *Red blood cells* are stored at 2–6°C for 35 days. They must be returned to the fridge within 30 minutes. They require a filtered transfusion administration set.

- *Platelets* are kept at 20–24°C for five days in the laboratory and gently agitated. Transfusion must be commenced as soon as possible. They require a special platelet administration set.
- *Fresh frozen plasma* can be kept at minus 30°C for two years. It is thawed in the laboratory by blood bank staff. Infusion should be started immediately once the plasma is thawed.

PREPARATION AND ADMINISTRATION

Some clinical areas require two trained staff to undertake preparation and administration, while other trusts may require one trained member of staff to perform this clinical skill. This trained and competent staff member must be a:

- doctor
- registered nurse
- nursing associate
- registered midwife
- operating department practitioner.

Students can often check as a third person, but cannot sign any of the paperwork.

The checker(s) should:

- check the patient's identification details against the blood unit, transfusion record and compatibility report form
- check the documentation: prescription, consent, reason for transfusion and baseline observations on the observation chart
- check the product issue: blood group, Rhesus D, blood bag number, blood unit, compatibility label, compatibility form
- check the product integrity and special requirements: leaks, clots, discoloration, expiry date, irradiation, CMV-negative, etc.

PRODUCT SPECIFICATIONS

Figure 14.2 shows a bag of blood group O Rh D-negative blood, which is also labelled as CMV-negative.

Blood is now traced from the vein of the donor to vein of the recipient and the barcodes on the bag represent the audit trial. The National Blood Transfusion Service uses a Pulse tracking system. All donors are given a unique donation number.

If the blood is not special blood, then we see a red block with 'not irradiated' on the bag. If a unit is irradiated then we would see a black block on the bag.

A blood transfusion record must be completed, including the compatibility form we brought back from the laboratory. This is the form that was attached to the first unit of blood to be transfused.

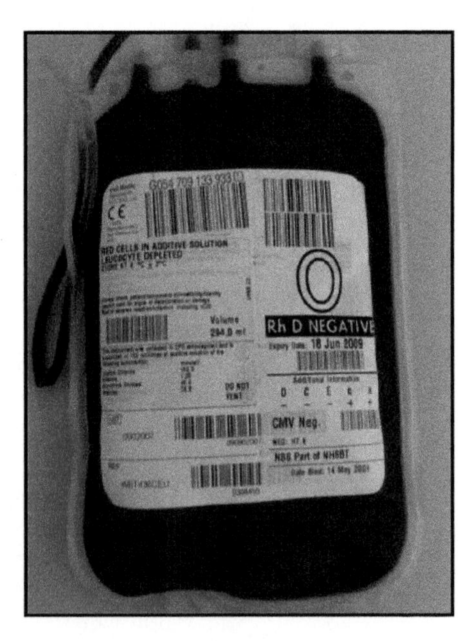

Figure 14.2 Blood bag. Source: Permission to reproduce this image is granted by North Bristol NHS Trust and University Hospitals Bristol NHS Foundation Trust.

PRE-TRANSFUSION CHECK

This bedside check is the last one. The patient should give verbal confirmation, checking all the details against the documentation and unit of blood. This compatibility document should be attached to the blood transfusion record sheet.

ADMINISTRATION PROCEDURE

The 'luggage label' is peeled off and attached to a ward register (after signing). Pathology laboratories usually store the originals of this paperwork as, legally, they must be kept for 30 years. The laboratories will then know where there blood went, as an extra check. Even if the patient received just a few drops from the transfusion, all this paperwork needs to be completed.

Remember to record the start time and unit volume on a fluid chart for your patient and *never* add any drugs to a bag of blood. The rate of transfusion should be monitored, as per the prescription.

The filtered blood/platelet administration set should be changed within 12 hours.

The end of the transfusion should be recorded on the compatibility report form and the observation chart. The empty blood bag should be retained for 24 hours, in case of any adverse reaction.

We may need to work out a drip rate manually, and will therefore need to know the formula for this, in case we cannot locate a machine for any reason. We will first need to know how many millilitres of fluid the bag contains and then the length of time that the prescription must take to go through (e.g. 450 ml and three hours). Blood administration sets deliver 15 drops per ml. This is the formula we use:

$$\text{Rate of transfusion} = \frac{\text{volume}}{\text{time in hours}} \times \frac{\text{drops per millilitre}}{\text{60 minutes}}$$

So, we have:

$$\frac{540\text{ ml}}{3\text{ hours}} \times \frac{15\text{ drops per ml}}{60\text{ minutes}} = 37.5\text{ drops per minute}$$

This is 450 divided by 3 multiplied by 15 divided by 60. Let a calculator do the work for you. This means that to get the bag of blood through in the prescribed time, we need to set the drip rate to 38 drops per minute.

MONITORING PROCEDURE

When the blood or blood product has been started, the patient must be watched while the first few millilitres are administered. We are looking for any adverse reactions.

The patient should be informed that they must report any shivering, pain, rash, flushing, anxiety, shortness of breath or generally feeling unwell.

Blood transfusion observations are performed *before* the transfusion, *within 15 minutes* of the transfusion going through and at the *end* of the transfusion. This is for every bag or product being transfused. We need to record:

- temperature
- pulse
- blood pressure
- respiratory rate.

Unconscious patients and patients being transfused need to be monitored more regularly.

Staff who can monitor the patient during the procedure include:

- doctor/clinical site manager
- registered nurse/midwife
- nursing associate
- operating department practitioner/assistant
- assistant practitioner

- student nurse/midwife/operating department practitioner or trainee assistant practitioner
- Band 3 healthcare assistant.

WHAT TO DO IF THE PATIENT EXPERIENCES AN ADVERSE REACTION

If there is a one degree C rise in the patient's temperature, *stop transfusion immediately*.

- Contact a doctor.
- Check the compatibility label with the patient's identification band.
- Record a full set of observations.
- Reassure the patient.
- Record the adverse reaction in the patient notes.

If transfusion is discontinued by a medic:

- the reaction must be reported to the blood bank
- a transfusion reaction form and an accident and incident management system (AIMS) form must be completed.

The medic may prescribe antihistamines and paracetamol, and may recommence with the transfusion, but at a slower rate.

SAFETY

For safety reasons, routine blood transfusions used to be administered between the hours of 08:00 and 20:00. This is because there were more staff on duty to observe for any adverse reactions during the daytime, and visible signs such as rashes are easier to spot in daylight. Today, however, blood is now administered 24/7.

TEST YOUR KNOWLEDGE

1. What observations need to be carried out for a blood transfusion and when?
2. What is a clinical indicator that the patient is having an adverse reaction to the transfusion?
3. How many blood components were issued in 2020?
4. What are the four blood services of the UK?
5. What is 'cryo'?
6. What does IBCT mean, in relation to blood transfusion errors?

KEY POINTS

- Understanding blood groups.
- Blood transfusion errors
- Blood transfusion documents and information leaflets.
- Blood collection procedures.
- Cold-chain requirements.
- Product specifications.
- Pre- and post-transfusion checks.

USEFUL WEB RESOURCES

NHS Blood and Transport. Give blood: www.blood.co.uk

Serious Hazards of Transfusion: www.shot.uk.org

NHS England. Blood transfusion: https://www.nhs.uk/conditions/blood-transfusion

National Institute for Health and Care Excellence. *Blood Transfusion*. NICE Guideline NG24: www.nice.org.uk/guidance/NG24

REFERENCE

SHOT (2021). *Annual SHOT Report 2020*. Manchester: Serious Hazards of Transfusion Available at https://www.shotuk.org/shot-reports.

Chapter 15

BASIC LIFE SUPPORT

Clinical Skills for Nurses, Second Edition. Claire Boyd.

LEARNING OUTCOMES

By the end of this chapter, you will have an understanding of the theory and practice of providing basic life support in the community and hospital settings.

Cardiopulmonary arrest can occur at any time and in any place. You will be given training in basic life support during your mandatory and statutory training programme in your induction to the work environment. You will learn during these sessions about the recovery position and jaw thrust, chin lift and how to use a 'stand back!' automated external defibrillator (AED).

DID YOU KNOW?

Cardiac arrest and heart attacks are not the same thing. A heart attack is when the blood flow to the heart is blocked. This blockage may initially cause chest pain and damage to some of the muscle to the heart. This may then trigger a cardiac arrest, when the heart actually stops pumping. This is why it is so important to recognise chest pain and give prompt treatment to reduce the risk of cardiac arrest.

This chapter is a guide to in-hospital adult and paediatric basic life support, based on the Resuscitation Council (UK) guidelines. It is aimed at healthcare professionals who are first to respond to an in-hospital cardiac arrest. We also look at those dealing with cardiac arrest in the community setting using an AED. However, before we begin, a mention of the ReSPECT initiative should be mentioned.

ReSPECT

ReSPECT stands for Recommended Summary Plan for Emergency Care and Treatment. In short, a plan stating what should happen if a person needs healthcare or treatment in an emergency, perhaps at a time when they are unable to make or express choices. These recommendations are created through conversation between a person, their family and their health and care professionals to understand what matters to them and what is realistic in terms of their care and treatment. The person's preferences and clinical recommendations are then recorded on a non-legally binding form, which can be reviewed and adapted if circumstances change.

The ReSPECT process is used in parts of the community and hospital settings, but not everywhere in the UK. It has increasing relevance for people who have complex health needs, people who are likely to be nearing the end of their lives, and people who are at risk of sudden deterioration or cardiac arrest.

In short, not everyone wants to be resuscitated.

SUMMONING HELP

In the acute hospital environment, many areas have four cardiac arrest teams that respond to emergency calls:

- adult
- paediatric (children less than 16years of age)
- maternal (pregnant women)
- neonatal.

You will need to know how to summon emergency assistance in your area; that is, what the call number is (often 2222) and the line of order (team dynamics) within the emergency responders. You should also familiarise yourself with the resuscitation trolley, perhaps by getting involved in the daily or weekly checks of this equipment and the emergency drug box. You should certainly be aware of where to find the defibrillator and all the emergency equipment, as it may be you who is asked to be the 'runner' who collects anything required by the emergency team.

Those in community settings without a cardiac arrest team will need to dial 999 for an ambulance, detailing the nature of the incident and performing basic life support until help arrives.

Whichever setting you work in, you need to be aware of whether a patient has legal documentation stating 'do not attempt cardiopulmonary resuscitation' (CPR) in their medical notes. It is ultimately the consultant's responsibility to arrange this legal notice. Other documentation to be aware of is the paperwork recorded after an in-hospital event. This is part of the standardised data collected by the National Cardiac Arrest Audit as part of an audit and quality-improvement process.

DID YOU KNOW?

Dialling 999, 112 or 911 will all connect you to 999 services in the UK.

THE DEBRIEF

After any emergency event, such as a cardiac arrest, it is good practice for staff to debrief. This will give everyone a chance to state what went well with the procedure and what did not go quite so well; this feedback is vital to improve everyone's performance in emergency events.

Patients who witnessed the flurry of activity surrounding an emergency event may be quite distressed, so some kind words, reassurance and perhaps a cup of tea will go a long way towards settling them.

CHAIN OF SURVIVAL

The Resuscitation Council (UK) has developed the chain of survival to aid us in increasing an individual's chances of survival (Figure 15.1).

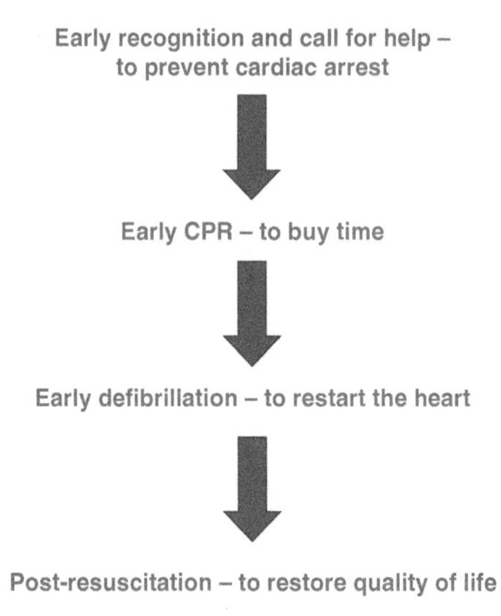

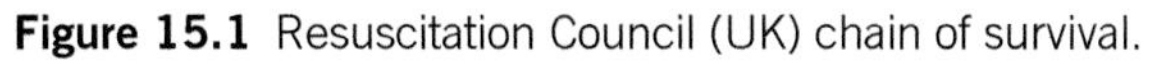

Figure 15.1 Resuscitation Council (UK) chain of survival.

AUTOMATED EXTERNAL DEFIBRILLATOR

Acute hospital settings may have defibrillators in every clinical area; they are also being seen increasingly in the community setting. Training is given to staff to use these generally larger machines.

Portable AEDs for use in the community are generally a much more simple affair. These devices have usually been purchased by organisations, including charities, local businesses, schools, gyms, dental surgeries, and are available for public access. Wherever they are found, they are intended to save the life of someone who has had a cardiac arrest. In short, AEDs are portable electronic machines that can automatically detect the abnormal heart rhythms that cause cardiac arrest and can deliver the shock needed to save the life of a person with a rhythm such as VF. Figure 15.2 shows a community AED, which are brightly coloured boxes affixed outside shops etc.

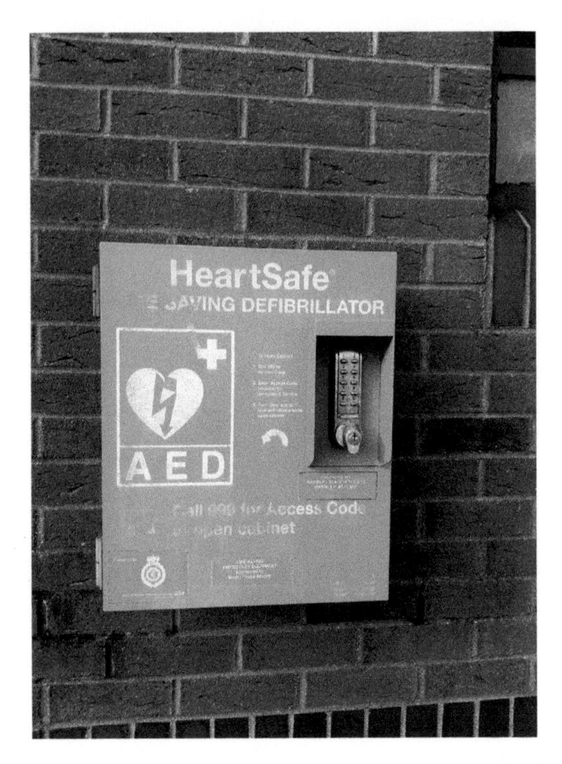

Figure 15.2 Community automated external defibrillator.

As these portable AEDs are used by the general public, they are very simple to use. To use the AED:

1. Recognise that someone who has collapsed, is unresponsive and not breathing normally is likely to have had a cardiac arrest.
2. Attach the two adhesive pads (electrodes) that connect the AED to the persons chest.
3. Switch on the AED machine.
4. Follow the instructions given by the AED machine.

To find where these AEDs are located in the community, there is a national list (see the web resources at the end of this chapter).

RESPONDING TO AN EMERGENCY EVENT (HOSPITAL SETTING)

The Collapsed Adult Patient

- On finding a collapsed patient or witnessing a collapse, we must first ensure our own personal safety and then immediately shout for help.
- We then need to check the patient for a response. This is done by gently shaking their shoulders and asking loudly 'Are you all right?'

The Responsive Patient

- If the patient responds, obtain an urgent medical assessment: this may be from the resuscitation team.
- While waiting for the medical assessment, administer oxygen therapy and assess the patient using the ABCDE approach and attach monitoring to record vital signs; for example, pulse oximetry, electrocardiogram (ECG), blood pressure (see Chapters 3 and 16).
- Obtain venous access.
- Hand over to the team using the SBAR (situation, background, assessment, recommendation) communication tool (see Chapter 3).

The following is the procedure for in-hospital resuscitation in the responsive patient and the collapsed/sick patient:

- Shout for HELP and assess patient.
- Signs of life? Yes.
- Assess ABCDE.
- Recognise and treat: oxygen, monitoring, intravenous access.
- Call resuscitation team, if appropriate.
- Hand over to the resuscitation team.

The Unresponsive Patient

- Shout for help again (if this has not already been done).
- Turn the patient on their back and open the airway using the head tilt and chin-lift technique. If you

suspect a cervical spine injury then use only the jaw thrust to open the airway. An airway adjunct may be inserted.

- Quickly listen, look and feel to determine whether the patient is breathing normally. This is performed by listening at the victim's mouth for breath sounds, looking for chest movement and feeling for air on your cheek.
- Listen for agonal breathing: this is when we hear occasional gasps and slow, laboured or noisy breathing, and is common immediately after a cardiac arrest. It should not be taken as a sign of life.
- More experienced staff may feel for a carotid pulse.

The Patient Has a Pulse or Other Signs of Life

- Urgent medical assessment is required. While waiting for the assessment, administer oxygen therapy and assess the patient using the ABCDE approach and attach monitoring to record vital signs (e.g. pulse oximetry, ECG, blood pressure (see Chapters 3 and 16).
- Obtain venous access.
- Hand over to the team using the SBAR communication tool (see Chapter 10).

The Patient Does Not Have a Pulse or Other Signs of Life

- One person starts CPR, one person calls the resuscitation team and one person collects the resuscitation equipment and a defibrillator. If only one person is present at this time, this will mean leaving the patient.
- Give 30 chest compressions followed by 2 ventilations.
- The correct hand position for chest compressions is the middle of the lower half of the sternum and the depth of the compressions should be 5–6 cm at a rate of at least 100–120 compressions each minute. The chest should recoil completely between each compression.
- The person providing chest compressions should change every two minutes, to avoid fatigue. This switch

should be conducted with the minimum amount of disruption to compressions.

- The airway should be maintained and the lungs ventilated. An airway adjunct may be placed in situ and a bag mask may be used for this ventilation, according to local policy, with supplemental oxygen therapy. If mouth-to-mouth ventilation is not commencing, continue with chest compressions until help or airway equipment arrives.
- When the defibrillator arrives, apply the self-adhesive pads to the patient, while still continuing with the chest compressions. Only those trained to use the defibrillator may use these machines and may defibrillate if appropriate.
- Advanced life support: when resuscitation team arrive. Hand over to the resuscitation team leader using the SBAR communication tool.
- Once sufficient staff are present, you may be required to prepare intravenous cannulation and/or any drugs required by the resuscitation team.

This is the in-hospital resuscitation procedure for the unresponsive patient:

1. Collapsed/sick patient.
2. Shout for HELP and assess patient.
3. Signs of life? No.
4. Call resuscitation team.
5. CPR compression/ventilation ratio 30 : 2 with oxygen and airway adjuncts.
6. Apply pads/monitor. Attempt defibrillation if appropriate.
7. Advanced life support when resuscitation team arrives.

Respiratory Arrest: If the Patient Is Not Breathing but Has a Pulse

Ventilate the patient's lungs and check for a pulse every 10 breaths. Only those competent in assessing breathing and a pulse will be able to make the diagnosis of respiratory arrest, so start chest compressions if there is any doubt about the presence of a pulse. Continue until more experienced help arrives.

THE PHONETIC ALPHABET

We have already discussed the SBAR communication tool, but during fraught moments our verbalisation may become a little garbled. When we put out an emergency call we need to have complete clarity in informing the emergency team of the exact location of the event. To do this, we might use the phonetic alphabet. For example, we may need the resuscitation team to come to 'D for Delta Ward'. The phonetic alphabet can be seen in Table 15.1.

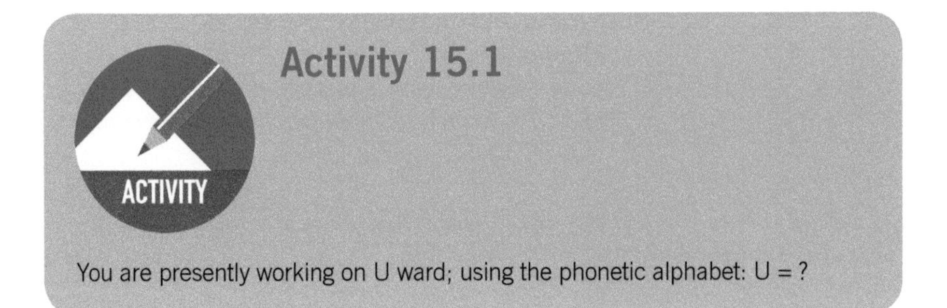

Activity 15.1

You are presently working on U ward; using the phonetic alphabet: U = ?

PAEDIATRIC BASIC LIFE SUPPORT

The Resuscitation Council (UK) states that many children receive no resuscitation because many rescuers fear that they will cause harm, as they have received no paediatric resuscitation training. However, research tells us that performing either chest compressions or expired air ventilation may result in a better outcome than doing nothing at all. Arrests of cardiac origin are seen predominantly in adults, while it is the asphyxial arrests that occur more commonly in children. Therefore a separate paediatric procedure has been devised, of two rescue breaths and 15 compressions (but starting with five rescue breaths), giving

Table 15.1 The NATO phonetic alphabet.

Letter	Phonetic	Letter	Phonetic
A	Alpha	N	November
B	Bravo	O	Oscar
C	Charlie	P	Papa
D	Delta	Q	Quebec
E	Echo	R	Romeo
F	Foxtrot	S	Sierra
G	Golf	T	Tango
H	Hotel	U	Uniform
I	India	V	Victor
J	Juliet	W	Whiskey
K	Kilo	X	X-Ray
L	Lima	Y	Yankee
M	Mike	Z	Zulu

us a CPR compression/ventilation ratio of 2:15. Chest-compression depths are at 4cm for infants and 5cm for children, with the rate being the same as for adult basic life support: 100compressions per minute, but not greater than 120compressions per minute. The recommended compression–ventilation ratio for newborn babies is 3:1.

This is the procedure for paediatric basic life support:

1. Unresponsive?
2. Shout for help.
3. Open airway.
4. Not breathing normally?
5. Five rescue breaths.
6. No sign of life?
7. Give 15 chest compressions.
8. CPR compression/ventilation ratio: 2 rescue breaths to 15 compressions.
9. Call resuscitation team.

RESPONDING TO AN EMERGENCY EVENT (COMMUNITY SETTING – USING AN AUTOMATED EXTERNAL DEFIBRILLATOR)

1. Recognise emergency situation. Check your environment for danger. Is the person responsive or unresponsive? If they respond – leave them in the position you found them and check whether they need any help. Reassess frequently.
2. If they are unresponsive, gently shake their shoulders for a response and ask if they are all right. Turn the person on to their back.
3. Airway – open airway.
4. Breathing – look, listen and feel (for no more than 10 seconds).
5. Alert others to your situation – shouting for help. Shout for the defibrillator (AED).
6. Dial 999. The 999 call handler will ask questions, stay on the line and give directions.
7. Start chest compressions: compress the chest at a rate of 100–120 compressions per minutes to a depth of 5–6 cm.
8. Use the AED – turn the machine on, apply pads on chest and follow prompts.
9. Note: if the ambulance is delayed, it is recommended to include rescue breaths. CPR ratio is 30 compressions to 2 ventilations.

TEST YOUR KNOWLEDGE

1. What is the chest compression/ventilation ratio for an adult?
2. At what depth should these compressions be?
3. What is the chest compression/ventilation ratio for an infant?
4. At what depth should these compressions be?
5. At what rate should the compressions be given for an adult?

6. At what rate should the compressions be given for a child?
7. In the phonetic alphabet, what word represents K?
8. What is a AED?
9. What does ReSPECT stand for?
10. In the phonetic alphabet, what word represents W?

KEY POINTS

- Adult basic life support.
- The phonetic alphabet.
- Paediatric basic life support.
- AED.

USEFUL WEB RESOURCES

Resuscitation Council UK: www.resus.org.uk
ReSPECT (Resuscitation Council UK): https://www.resus.org.uk/respect
National Defibrillator Database: https://www.nddb.uk

Chapter 16

PERFORMING AN ELECTROCARDIOGRAM

LEARNING OUTCOMES

By the end of this chapter you will have an understanding of the theory and practice of performing the clinical skill of recording an electrocardiogram (ECG).

An ECG is a diagnostic test that measures the electrical activity and muscular functions of the heart from electrodes that have been placed on the patient's chest and limbs. These electrodes transmit the electrical impulses generated by the heart to the ECG machine; the machine then produces a graph, called the ECG tracing. These results show the rate and rhythm of the heartbeat, as well as providing indirect evidence of the blood flow to the heart muscle. The top two chambers of the heart and the bottom two chambers of the heart contract and relax together, smoothly. The heart muscle is like an elastic band pulling and bouncing back. This contraction depends on the electrical charge. The ECG tells us if there is any blockages with this electrical charge.

Patients may ask about the possibility of getting an electrical shock from the procedure, but you can reassure them that it is not dangerous because no electricity is sent through the body. There is no risk of electrical shock and an ECG is painless.

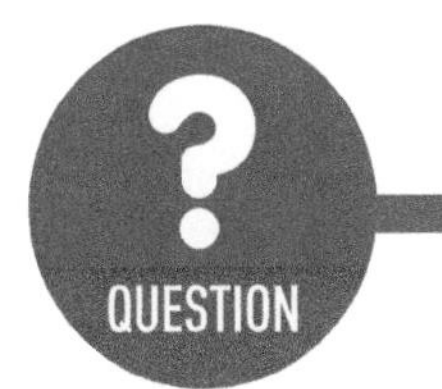

Question 16.1 Why do we call the ECG machine a '12-lead ECG' when in actual fact it has only 10 leads?

A standard ECG machine has 10 leads to attach to 10 electrodes on the body, which actually produces **12 electrical views of the heart**; this is why we call the machine a 12-lead ECG. Figure 16.1 shows a typical ECG machine.

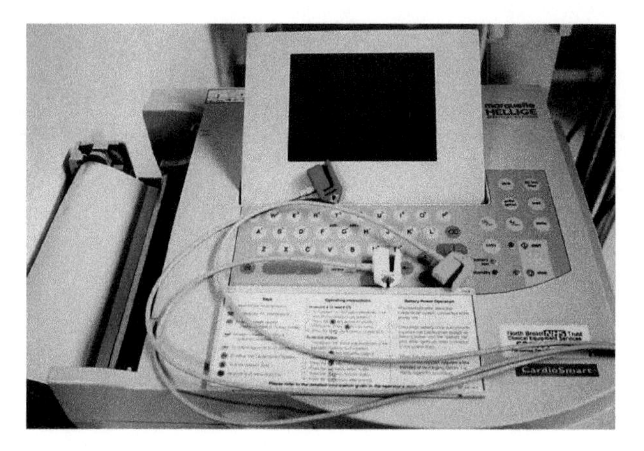

Figure 16.1 An ECG machine.

An electrode is placed on each arm and leg and the remaining six are placed across the chest wall. It is important to have training for the machine in use in your area.

There are many reasons why a doctor will request an ECG recording on an individual, but very often you will just use your use intuition to perform this skill (i.e. not waiting to be asked to perform an ECG) as you become more experienced. An ECG might be performed:

- when a patient is experiencing chest pain – possibly a myocardial infarction (MI; this is where blood is not received in the heart muscle, a heart attack; an area of the heart dies)
- when there is an arrhythmia – the pulse is not regular
- routinely – baseline on admission – checking for any abnormalities
- post-MI
- when the patient has chest pain from ischaemia – ischaemia is a reduced blood supply to the heart
- before and after insertion of a pacemaker – which keeps the heart regular

- Where there is hypo- or hypertension – the patient's blood pressure is low or high if messages are not getting through to the heart (blocked or interrupted)
- preoperatively – diagnostic to establish whether the patient is fit enough to undergo surgery
- in cases of syncope – (a posh word for fainting/ dizziness). The patient should have lying and standing blood pressure recordings taken. If our blood pressure is low we may feel faint.
- when a pulmonary embolism is causing strain to the heart
- when the patient has breathing difficulties – again putting a strain on the heart
- if a patient is experiencing vacant episodes, possibly due to low blood glucose (hypoglycaemia)
- in cases of stroke
- in cases of seizure.

BASIC ANATOMY OF THE HEART

The heart has four chambers: the right and left atria and the right and left ventricles. The right side of the heart collects blood from the body and pumps it to the lungs, whereas the left side of the heart receives the blood from the lungs and pumps it to the body. Like all muscles and cells, the heart requires oxygen and nutrients to function; these are supplied by arteries that originate from the aorta.

The heart contains specialised cells that initiate and conduct electrical impulses. This conduction system is shown in Figure 16.2.

Electrically, the heart can be divided into upper and lower chambers: the heartbeat *originates* in the sinoatrial (SA) node. This node acts independently of the brain to generate electricity for the heart to beat; it is often referred to as the automatic pacemaker. The rate at which the SA node fires is dependent on the vagus nerve: an increase in vagal activity *slows* the heart rate and a decrease in vagal activity *speeds up* the heart rate.

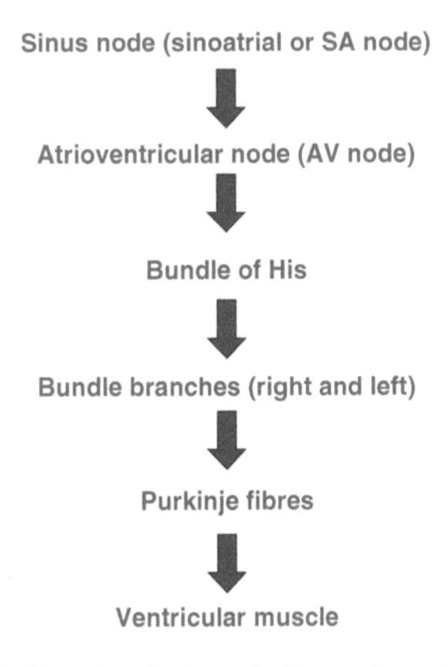

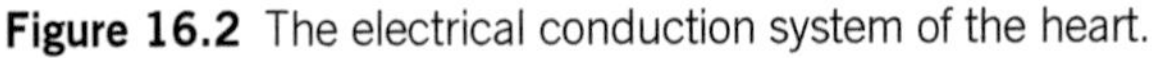

Figure 16.2 The electrical conduction system of the heart.

Atropine is used to block the vagus nerve when we need to increase the heart rate.

The SA node fires and the electrical impulse spreads across the atria causing atrial contraction: the **P wave**. This electrical impulse stimulates the atria to squeeze and push blood into the ventricles of the heart (known as myocardial contractions). As this is happening, the impulse is slowed down, presenting as a straight line (isoelectric line) between the end of the P wave and the beginning of the QRS complex.

The electrical impulse progresses to the atrioventricular (AV) node down to the bundle of His and then through the right and left bundle branches and ending in the Purkinje fibres, which stimulates the ventricles to contract to pump blood to the body and lungs. The septum (dividing wall) is depolarised from left to righ,t with the left ventricle exerting more influence than the right. This ventricular depolarisation and contraction produces the **QRS complex**. The ventricles then repolarize: this is the **T wave**. Figure 16.3 shows how the P wave, QRS complex and T wave are presented on an ECG recording.

GLOSSARY

Heart muscles contract or relax depending on the electrical charge:

Depolarisation

Part of heart contracting or pushing blood down into the bottom chambers from the top chambers (i.e. emptying)

Repolarisation

The bottom two chambers of the heart relax and fill up with blood.

DID YOU KNOW?

P waves = atrial contraction
QRS complex = ventricular contractions
T waves = repolarisation of ventricles
PR interval = time after atria contract until ventricles contract
ST segment = time for repolarisation and recovery

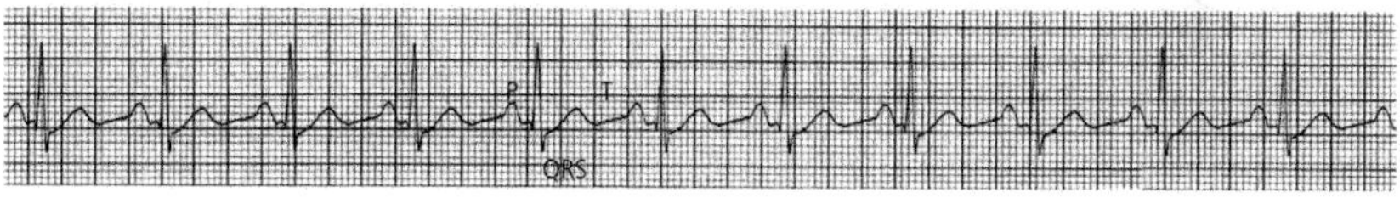

Figure 16.3 The ECG and its relation to cardiac contraction (Jevon, 2010).

ECG PAPER AND SPEED

The ECG paper speed is ordinarily **25 mm per second.** As a result, each 1 mm (small) horizontal box corresponds to 0.04 second, with heavier lines forming larger boxes that include five small boxes and hence represent 0.2 seconds intervals; 1 big square = 5 small squares.

One small square (1 mm) = 0.04 seconds

One large square (5 mm) = 0.2 seconds

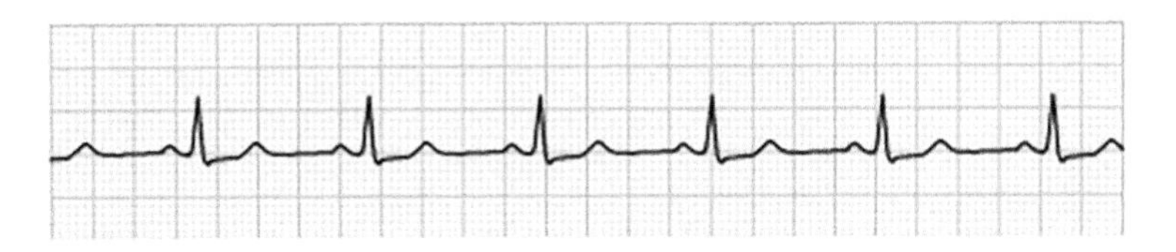

Figure 16.4 Sinus rhythm.

Five large squares (25 mm) = 1 second

You may wish to view Figure 16.4, which shows the sinus rhythm, to see the ECG paper.

THE PROCEDURE

Before the ECG can be recorded there are various items of equipment that need to be gathered:

- the ECG machine
- a disposable razor
- tissues
- alcohol wipes
- 10 disposable pre-gelled electrodes (check expiry date, as dry gel inhibits conduction)
- gloves (if there is any possibility of contamination with blood or other bodily fluids).

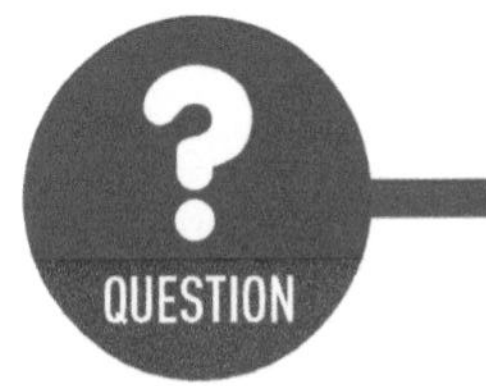

Question 16.2 What position should a patient be in for an ECG recording?

Pull the curtains around the bed space for privacy and dignity and gain consent. Patients will then be asked to remove upper clothing and lie semi-recumbent.

Women will need to remove their bras. Some patients may require assistance to undress. Some patients will be unable to lie semi-recumbent or flat so may need to sit in a chair for this procedure. In these cases, the patient should not sit higher than 45 degrees; this should be recorded on the tracing. It is important to keep the patient warm to reduce muscle tremor (shivering). Explain the procedure to the patient, keeping them well informed.

PERFORMING THE ECG

1. Wash your hands before and after the procedure.
2. Unless it is an emergency situation, consent should be gained before the procedure can start.
3. Ensure that the bed is at a comfortable height for performing the procedure.
4. Once you are sure that the patient is comfortable, informed and warm, you can start the ECG recording.
5. To ensure good contact, if the skin is greasy, wipe it with a 70% isopropyl alcohol swab and then dry the area with clean gauze. If you place the electrode on wet alcohol, it will adversely affect the trace. Place the pre-gelled electrode over the swabbed area. If the skin is not greasy, you can apply the pre-gelled electrode directly to the skin.
6. If the patient has excess chest hair, it may need removing. Most pre-gelled tabs do stick to the skin despite the hairs; you will have to use your own judgement or, if you are not sure, ask a more experienced member of staff for advice. If clipping is required (shaving is not recommended for infection control reasons) the patient may feel more comfortable clipping himself. If you have to clip the patient, be careful they have any skin blemishes or spots and be vigilant when clipping around the nipple area. Also, if necessary, take into consideration the patient's cultural background; gain permission and consent before clipping either chest or limb hair.
7. If the skin is wet, dry the area before applying the electrode.
8. It is important to remember that correct lead placement is essential and the tabs should be placed in the same (correct) place for each individual recording. If the patient has abnormal anatomy (i.e. kyphoscoliosis) then you should still follow the same principles, using the ribs as guides, as the trace can be replicated when necessary.

9. If the patient has eczema, psoriasis or other skin conditions that may prevent correct lead placement, place the tabs as close to the correct area as possible, record the trace and document clearly why there was abnormal lead placement.
10. If you are recording a trace on a patient with large breasts, the general rule is to make an assessment as to the easiest access to the rib spaces. If access is easiest by placing the tabs under the breast, that is fine, or if access to the rib space is easiest on top of the breast, then that is fine as well. You will have to make your own assessment and use your own judgement.

PLACEMENT OF THE LEADS

The leads should be placed in specific positions, and you will need to familiarise yourself with them during your training in this clinical procedure.

Limb Leads

Ride Your Green Bike

Limb leads are often colour coded; the colours used may vary by manufacturer of the ECG machine, so do check. Many are red, yellow, green and blue, so nurses tend to say 'ride your green bike' as a reminder for lead/electrode placement. But each lead can be identified by the following abbreviations.

RA: right arm/right wrist

LA: left arm/left wrist

RL: right leg/ankle

LL: left leg/ankle

Note: Limb leads can be put on the shoulders and thighs if necessary.

Chest Leads

C1: fourth intercostal space, right sternal border.

C2: fourth intercostal space, left sternal border.

C3: midway between C2 and C4.

C4: fifth intercostal space, left midclavicular line.

C5: fifth intercostal space, left anterior axillary line.

C6: fifth intercostal space, left midaxillary line.

To obtain the midaxillary line, find the midline and come down – draw imaginary line.
Some machines have pictures when they are switched on to show where to place the tabs.

Five-lead ECG

Five-lead monitors may also be in use in many clinical areas.

These leads are placed as follows:

- right shoulder (RA)
- left shoulder (LA)
- fourth intercostal space (V1)
- right abdomen (RL)
- left abdomen (LL).

HEART MONITORS

A heart monitor (called cardiac monitoring) or defibrillation machine may be used for an ECG recording for patients who may require continuous cardiac monitoring, perhaps using a mobile transportable device, due to:

- chest pain
- post-MI

- arrhythmias or potential arrhythmias present
- starting a newly prescribed drug treatment
- having taken an overdose
- having abnormally low or high blood chemistry.

These machines have three leads and the electrodes are placed on the:

- right shoulder: this is the negative electrode
- left shoulder: this is the earth electrode
- left abdomen: this is the positive electrode.

These monitors only measure the rate and rhythm of the heartbeat, so this monitoring does not constitute a complete ECG. The electrodes are usually colour coded; you will need to familiarise yourself with the instructions for each particular machine and set of electrodes, as different machines and leads use different colour-coded tabs.

UNUSUAL CIRCUMSTANCES

As with any clinical skill, we should be prepared for the unusual when conducting an ECG, such as:

- Amputees – put a tab on the stump; tabs do not need to be equally placed on the body or matching.
- Skin conditions – rub off any creams/lotions otherwise tabs will not stick.
- Hypersensitivity to the tabs – use hypoallergenic tabs.
- Nipple rings – cover a ring with tape if you cannot remove it for any reason.
- Very hairy chest – remove hair.
- Parkinson's disease – includes rigours and other shakes, such as anxiety; putting on the 'filter on' switch does not eliminate this shaking on the tracing.
- Dextrocardia – this is where the heart is on the wrong side of the body – just adjust the tabs to be placed on the right side of the body instead of the left.

RECORDING

Once the electrodes have been attached to the patient and before the recording is obtained, and to get a good trace, the following should be addressed:

- Ask the patient to relax.
- Ask the patient to put both arms by their sides.
- Ask the patient to breathe gently (no need to hold their breath).
- Ask the patient not to talk during recording the trace.
- Ensure that the leads are tangle-free and not crossed.
- Check that the machine has been calibrated and that there is paper in the machine.

TRICKS OF THE TRADE

- Keep the patient warm – relaxed.
- Make sure that the appropriate person reviews the recording.
- Correct lead placement is essential – if leads need to be placed in 'incorrect' position – record this clearly.
- Don't fall into the trap of telling the patient, 'It looks OK'.

AFTERCARE

Once the recording has been completed, the patient may need help to remove the electrodes. Take care when removing them: if the patient has friable skin the removal of the electrode may cause trauma, so remove them carefully.

Check for signs of an allergic reaction. If allergic signs are present (redness, itchiness, soreness directly relating to electrode placement areas), inform the doctor and the patient. Record what you have seen.

If clinically indicated (e.g. acute chest pain or arrhythmia), the ECG tabs may need to stay in place (for serial recordings); if so, be careful when unhooking the leads from the tabs, trying not to disturb them.

The patient may become anxious following the procedure and may ask you what the ECG shows. Take care when answering; remember you are only *recording* and not *interpreting* the ECG, which is an advanced clinical skill.

Help the patient to get dressed, if necessary.

Note: not all ECGs are performed in a routine manner; ECGs are often needed in response to an emergency situation. Despite the urgency, the above principles must be adhered to. If a person is suffering from a cardiac-related condition, correct recording of the ECG is essential for helping the assessment and treatment of the patient.

DOCUMENTATION

Inform nursing and medical staff *immediately* that the recording has been obtained. If the machine does not record the patient's name automatically you will need to write the following on the tracing:

- the patient's name
- the patient's date of birth
- date of ECG
- time of ECG
- whether the filter setting was on or off
- the intensity of any chest pain that the patient is experiencing.

THE RECORDINGS

Sinus Rhythm

Figure 16.4 shows sinus rhythm. Sinus rhythm is the normal rhythm of the heart, which originates in the sinus node. This is what sinus rhythm means:

QRS rate	60–100 beats per minute
QRS rhythm	regular
QRS width	normal
P waves	present, normal, relationship between P waves and QRS complexes = P wave precedes each QRS complex.

Sinus Tachycardia

Sinus tachycardia means:

QRS rate	more than 100 beats per minute
QRS rhythm	regular
QRS width	normal
P waves	present, normal but more than 100 beats per minute; relationship between P waves and QRS complexes, P wave precedes each QRS complex.

ABNORMAL ECG RECORDINGS

You would expect to see abnormal ECG recordings, as in Table 16.1.

PROBLEMS WITH THE RECORDING

Sometimes problems may be encountered with an ECG recoding itself, some of which are outlined in Table 16.2.

Table 16.1 Abnormal ECG recordings.

Problem	Possible cause
Abnormal heart rhythms (arrhythmias)	**Heart valve disease**
Cardiac muscle defect	**Inflammation of the heart (myocarditis)**
Congenital heart defect	**Changes in the amount of electrolytes (chemicals in the blood)**
Coronary artery disease	**Past heart attack**
Ectopic heartbeat	**Present or impending heart attack**
Enlargement of the heart	**Slower-than-normal heart rate (bradycardia)**
Faster than normal heart rate (tachycardia)	**Interference on machine (i.e. 'electrical noise')**

Table 16.2 Problems that may be encountered with an ECG recording.

Problem	Solution
Straight line	Check the patient, then check the C2 lead. Asystole rarely produces a straight line.
Poor-quality ECG	Check all the connections and brightness display. Check that all electrodes are correctly attached. Ensure that the skin where the electrodes are placed is dry; wipe the skin with an alcohol swab if necessary.
Interference and artefacts	The causes may be poor electrode contact, patient movement and interference (possibly caused by infusion pumps). Apply electrodes over bone to remedy.
Wandering baseline	Usually caused by patient movement. Reposition electrodes away from the lower ribs.
Small ECG complexes	Could be caused by pericardial effusion, obesity and hypothyroidism. Could be a technical problem: check that the correct ECG monitoring leads have been selected.
Incorrect heart rate display	Results in small QRS complexes on the paper trace, possibly due to interference and muscle movement. Keep the patient warm.

INTERPRETATING THE RECORDING

This chapter has looked at how to record an ECG. Interpreting these recordings is a whole new skill. So, at first you may be asked to just take an ECG recording and show it to the appropriate personnel. But seven recordings are illustrated here:

- a shivering patient
- AC interference (artefact)
- a patient experiencing an MI
- arterial fibrillation (AF)
- ventricular fibrillation (VF)
- VT
- asystole.

A Shivering Patient

Figure 16.5 shows a reading from a shivering patient, which could be caused by the patient shivering from cold or due to:

- hypothermia
- Anxiety
- Parkinson's disease.

AC Interference (Artefact)

Figure 16.6 shows interference on the trace. This tracing shows: electrical interference; you will need to press filter

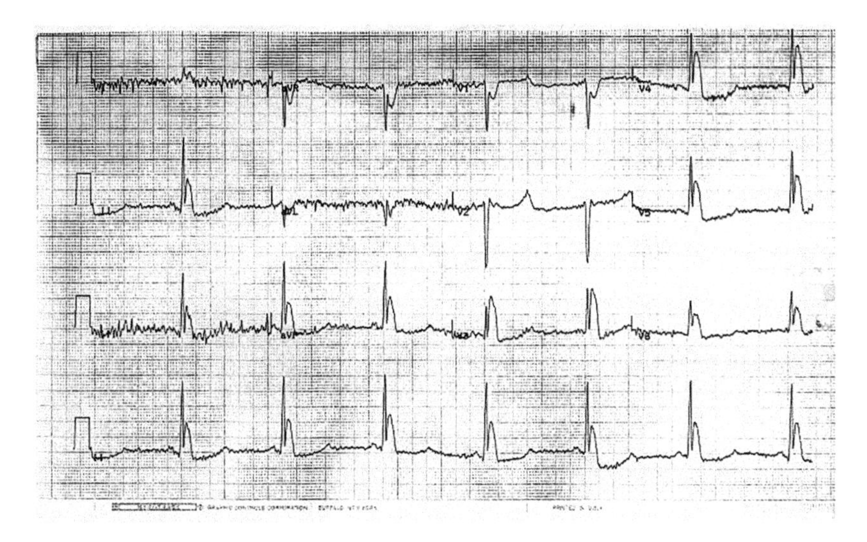

Figure 16.5 ECG tracing from a shivering patient.

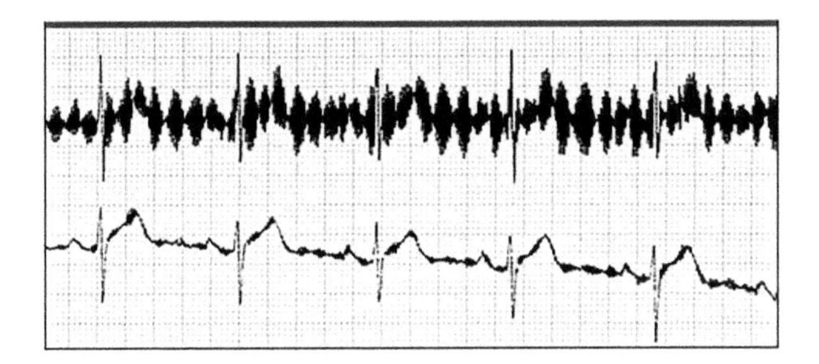

Figure 16.6 AC interference on an ECG trace.

button. **Check** to see whether any pumps or electrical equipment nearby can be turned off.

A Patient Experiencing a Myocardial Infarction

Figure 16.7 shows a patient experiencing an MI. The T wave should be positive but showing as negative.

Atrial Fibrillation

Figure 16.8 shows a patient experiencing atrial fibrillation (AF), while Table 16.3 shows the symptoms, causes and treatment of AF. This is the most common occurring arrhythmia you will see in clinical practice; there is reduced

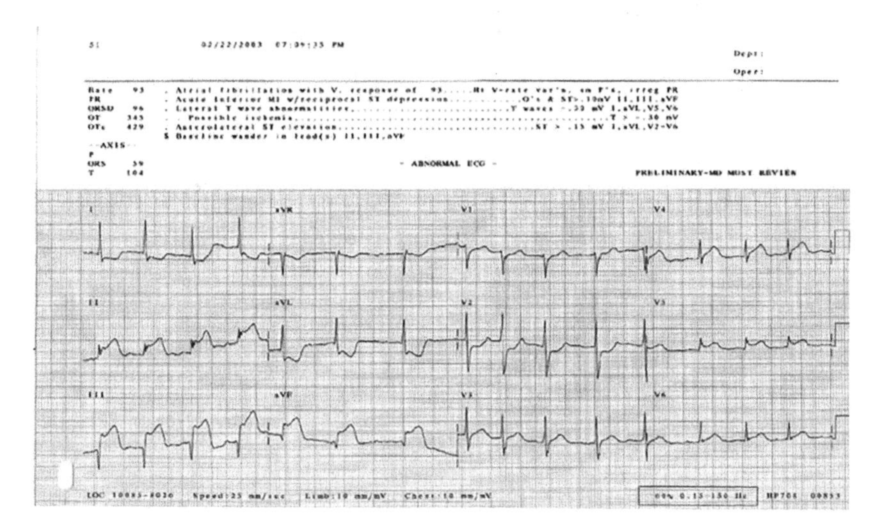

Figure 16.7 Typical trace of a patient experiencing a myocardial infarction.

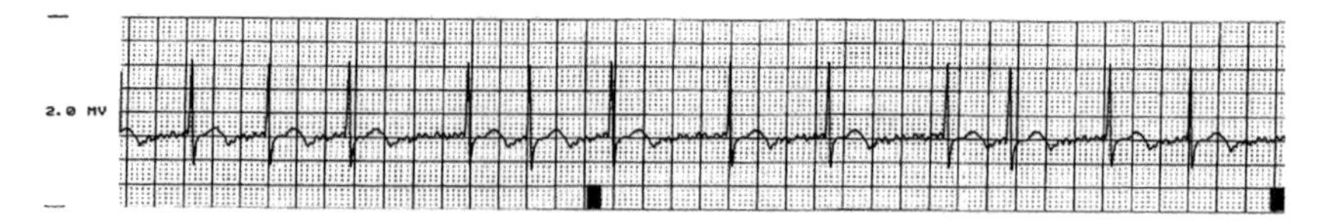

Figure 16.8 Atrial fibrillation.

Table 16.3 Symptoms, causes and treatment for atrial fibrillation.

Symptoms	Causes	Treatment
Palpitations	Hypertension	Flecainide
Dyspnoea	Hyperthyroidism	Amiodarone
Syncope/dizziness/light-headedness	Electrolyte imbalance	Digoxin
Fatigue	Pneumonia	Verapamil
Confusion	Pulmonary embolism	Cardioversion
Ischaemic chest pain	Myocarditis	Ablation

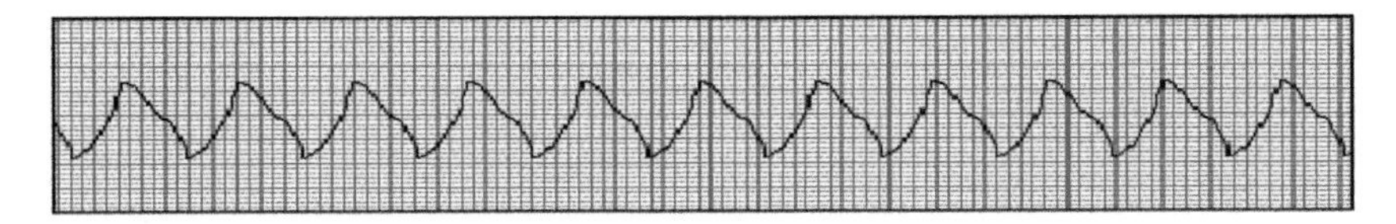

Figure 16.9 Ventricular fibrillation.

atrial 'kick' and reduced ventricular filling time, which leads to reduced cardiac output.

Ventricular Fibrillation

Ventricular fibrillation (VF) is defined as an erratic disorganised firing of impulses from the ventricles causing an inability to contract or pump blood to the body. Figure 16.9 shows VF on the tracing.

Ventricular Tachycardia

Ventricular tachycardia (VT) is a heart rhythm disorder (arrhythmia) caused by the abnormal electrical signals in the lower chambers of the heart ventricles. Figure 16.10 shows VT on the tracing.

Asystole

Asystole means 'absence of', in this case showing a cardiac arrest with no conduction activity. Figure 16.11 shows asystole on the tracing.

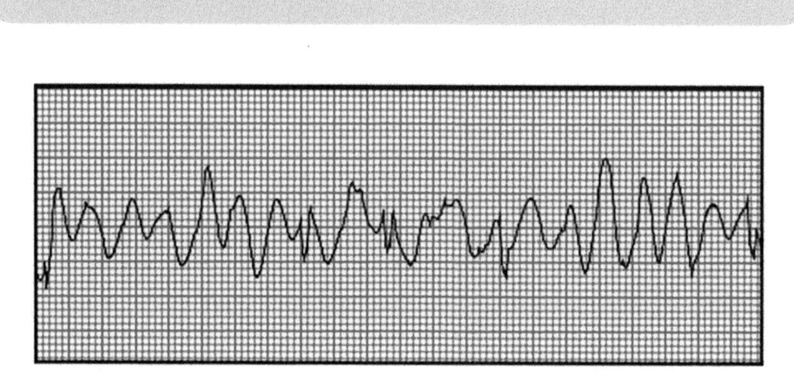

Figure 16.10 Ventricular tachycardia.

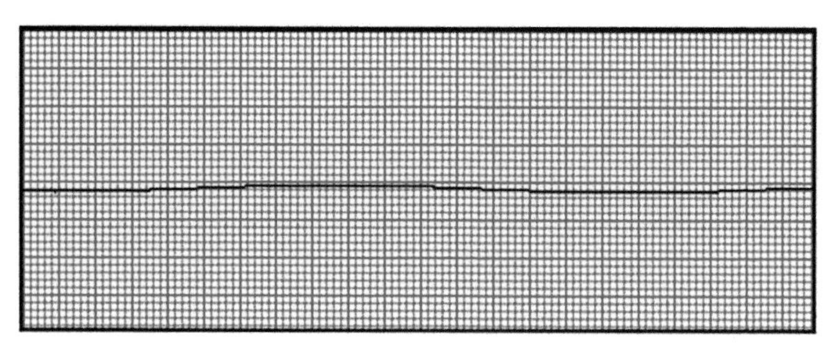

Figure 16.11 Asystole.

DID YOU KNOW?

- If PR interval is too long – this is a first-degree heart block.
- If PR is normal but beats are dropped – this is a second-degree heart block.
- If there is no relationship between P waves and QRS waves – this is a complete heart block.

TEST YOUR KNOWLEDGE

1 The normal recording speed of an ECG is:

A 33 mm per second.

B 25 mm per second.

- **C** 10 mm per second.
- **D** 60 mm per second.

2 AC interference is caused by:

- **A** low battery in the machine.
- **B** the patient having a pacemaker.
- **C** the patient talking during the recording.
- **D** electrical interference.

3 What do you need to ask the patient to do during the ECG procedure? Pick as many as apply.

- **A** Relax.
- **B** Not to talk during the procedure.
- **C** Sit upright.
- **D** Hold your breath.

4 What should you say to the patient after the recording?

- **A** 'It looks OK'.
- **B** 'Oh dear, poor you!'
- **C** 'I need to show the recording to the doctor; this is standard procedure'.
- **D** 'Do you want to keep the tracing?'

5 Asystole is a normal ECG recording.

- **A** True.
- **B** False.

6 The T wave should show as a positive on an ECG recording of someone experiencing a MI.

- **A** True.
- **B** False.

KEY POINTS

- The ECG machine.
- Heart monitors.
- Basic anatomy of the heart.
- Performing the ECG recording.

USEFUL WEB RESOURCES

NHS England. Electrocardiogram (ECG): https://www.nhs.uk/conditions/electrocardiogram

British National Formulary: https://bnf.nice.org.uk

REFERENCE

Jevon, P. (2010). *Advanced Cardiac Life Support: A guide for nurses*, 2e. Oxford: Wiley Blackwell.

Answers

CHAPTER 1

Activity 1.1

Clinical activity	Sterile gloves	Non-sterile gloves	Aseptic, ANTT or clean technique?
Providing mouth care to the unconscious patient		✓	Clean
Inserting a urinary catheter	✓		Aseptic
Preparing intravenous medications		✓	ANTT
Emptying a urinary catheter		✓	clean
Emptying a urinal full of urine		✓	Clean
Emptying a commode full of faeces		✓	Clean
Inserting a cannula into a patient's hand		✓	ANTT
Taking blood via venepuncture		✓	ANTT
Changing a tracheostomy stoma dressing	✓		Aseptic
Changing a surgical wound site	✓		Aseptic

Activity 1.2

Would you wear a non-sterile apron to perform these clinical tasks?

- Bed-bathing a patient – yes.
- Emptying a bed pan/urinal – yes.
- Making a bed – yes.
- Washing a bed – yes.
- Changing a stoma bag – yes.
- Cleaning a trolley – yes.
- Cleaning a drip stand – yes.
- Inserting a peripheral cannula – yes.

Clinical Skills for Nurses, Second Edition. Claire Boyd.

Test Your Knowledge

1. Asepsis is to be free from all pathogenic micro-organisms.
2. False.
3. No.
4. No.
5. Aseptic non-touch technique wearing non-sterile gloves.
6. Clean technique wearing non-sterile gloves.
7. Correct use of personal protective equipment.
8. True.
9. False – this is surgical aseptic non-touch technique.
10. Six links.

CHAPTER 2

Activity 2.1

Did you notice that it is only the systolic blood pressure recording that generates a score on the chart in the blood pressure section?

So, only the blood pressure of 202 mmHg generated a score, of 2.

Activity 2.2

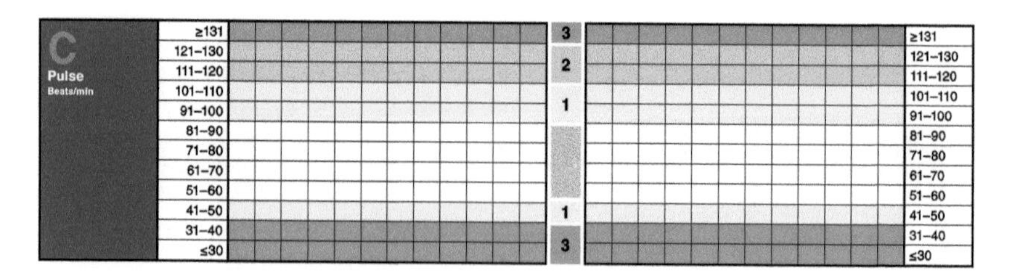

102 bpm generates a score of 1.

Activity 2.3

Cyanosis	Cyanosed/blue tinge to skin, lips, nail beds or in the mucous membrane (in mouth). Patients with anaemia may have insufficient haemoglobin to produce cyanotic appearance.
Blood gases	Increased carbon dioxide makes the blood values acidic. Increased oxygen makes the blood values alkaline. Respiratory acidosis occurs if pH is below 7.28 (likelihood of death).
Hypoxia	Lack of oxygen in the tissues.
Hypercapnia	Higher than normal levels of carbon dioxide in the bodily tissues.
Hypoxaemia	Decreased oxygen levels in arterial blood.
Tidal volume	The amount of air breathed in and out during a single breath (normally 500 ml).

Total lung capacity	The amount of air the lungs can hold is approximately 5–6 litres.
Residual volume	The volume of air remaining in the lungs at the end of a forceful expiration.

Questions

2.1 (i) To establish a baseline reading; (ii) to monitor fluctuations in temperature (i.e. fever), ovulation in women; (iii) to monitor signs of incompatibility during blood transfusion; (iv) to monitor the temperature of patients being treated for infection; (v) to monitor the temperature of patients recovering from hypothermia.

2.2 Temporal, common carotid, brachial, radial, femoral, popliteal, posterior tibial, dorsalis pedis. See Figure 2.5 for positions in the body.

Test Your Knowledge

1 NEWS 2 score = 8
- Respiratory rate: 30 breaths per minute = 3
- Oxygen saturation, SpO_2: 95% scale 1 supplementary oxygen = 2
- Blood pressure: 192/74 mmHg = 0
- Heart rate: 110 bpm = 2
- Neurological response: alert = 0
- Temperature: 38.4°C = 2

2 Tracheostomy mask.

3 A score of 3 in any single parameter directs us to continue monitoring the patient once hourly and to inform the nurse in charge and the doctor.

4 120–160 bpm.

5 OH = orthostatic hypotension.

6 New confusion.

Actions: continuous monitoring of vital signs:
- Registered nurse to immediately inform the medical team caring for the patient – this should be at least at specialist registrar level.
- Emergency assessment by a team with critical care competencies, including practitioner(s) with advanced airway management skills.
- Consider transfer of care facility (i.e. higher-dependency unit or intensive care).
- Clinical care in an environment with monitoring facilities.

CHAPTER 3

Activity 3.1

NEWS 2 values: respiratory rate = 2; SpO_2 = 2 + 0 = 2; blood pressure = 3; heart rate = 2; neurological response (ACVPU) = 3; temperature = 0; Total NEWS = 12.Action: recheck score. Inform nurse in charge. A total score of 7 or more directs us to obtain an emergency medical assessment.

Activity 3.2

Identify yourself and clinical area: 'Doctor, I'm concerned about Sandra Singh who underwent a bowel resection three days ago. I have just assessed her and her NEWS score is 12. I have administered oxygen via a non-rebreather mask. I will insert two peripheral cannulas and perform an ECG. Please review immediately.'Note: Two peripheral cannulas may be inserted during emergency situations. Did you notice that I just gave the NEWS score, as this is an emergency situation, to save vital time.

Questions

3.1 Oliguria: production of abnormally small amounts of urine; may be caused by conditions such as excessive sweating, kidney disease, loss of blood or diarrhoea.
Anuria: where the kidneys fail to produce urine or the output is less than 100 ml in 24 hours.
Absolute anuria: absence of urine output, generally reflecting a form of obstruction.

Test Your Knowledge

1. Situation, background, assessment, recommendation: a communication tool.
2. A = 2, B = 2, C (blood pressure) = 0, C (pulse) = 0, D = 0, E = 0. Total NEWS 2 = 4
3. Airway, breathing, circulation (cannulation), disability (neurological assessment) and diuresis (drugs and diabetes), exposure and early call for help using SBAR.
4. A measurement of the rate at which blood refills empty capillaries.

CHAPTER 4

Activity 4.1

a Deep yellow/orange urine could be due to dehydration or jaundice. Bilirubin – the breakdown product of haemoglobin, excreted in bile and in small amounts of urine – may be detected in a urinalysis test. It may also be caused by drugs such as rifampicin.

b Blue urine may be caused by a chemical (antimicrobial) called methylene blue, which is added to fresh frozen plasma (a blood product transfusion) and administered to neonates and small children. This chemical is added to inactivate any viruses present in this blood product to protect their underdeveloped immune systems. It may also cause temporarily blue skin, the reason why parents may call their baby a 'smurf baby'!

c Red urine may be blood caused by trauma or kidney cancer. It may also be caused by eating large amounts of beetroot, but this is only temporary.

d Blue/green urine may be caused by a pseudomonal urine infection. A urinalysis test would show protein in the urine.

Questions

4.1 Urine consists of 95% water + constituents shown in Table 4.1. Protein should not be present in urine.

Test Your Knowledge

1. The involuntary passing of urine.
2. Nocturnal enuresis.
3. Stress incontinence, urgency/urge incontinence, overflow inconti-

nence, reflex incontinence, environmental/locomotor incontinence, functional incontinence.

4 Meconium.

5 Usual stool consistency and frequency, pain associated with bowel motion, presence of blood and/or mucus, evacuation problems, past medical history, toilet access issues, diet and fluid intake, medication, including over-the-counter medications.

6 75% water and 25% solid matter.

7 Gluteal cleft or bottom crack.

8 Incontinence-associated dermatitis.

9 Pressure ulcer has a raised edge, Moisture lesion has a diffuse and irregular edge.

10 Skin assessment, continence assessment, nutritional assessment, falls and manual handling assessment.

CHAPTER 5

Activity 5.1

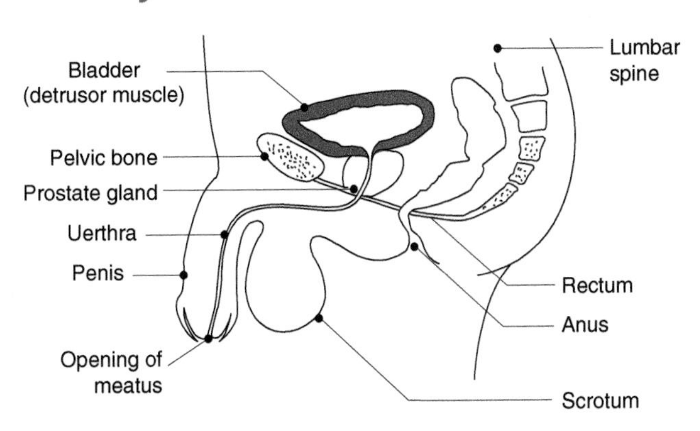

Permission to reproduce this image is granted by North Bristol NHS Trust and University Hospitals Bristol NHS Foundation Trust

Questions

5.1 A urethral stricture is damage to the urethral lining.

5.2 Priapism is a persistent and often painful erection that requires immediate decompression. It may be caused by local or spinal cord damage.

Test Your Knowledge

1 Clean intermittent (CIC), urethral (URC), suprapubic (SPC) catheterisation.

2 CIC: can give individuals independence and control over their own bodies; URC: suitable for most patients requiring bladder drainage; SPC: can be used if URC is unsuitable (i.e. due to trauma).

3 CIC, patients must have good dexterity and cognitive function to be able to self-care; URC, high risk of infection (catheter-associated urinary tract infection); SPC, contraindicated in patients with bladder tumours or unexplained haematuria.

4 Urethral trauma resulting in infection and possible septicaemia/renal failure/death; formation of false urethral passage; bladder perforation; traumatic removal of catheter with balloon inflated; urinary tract infection and possible septicaemia/renal failure/death; bypassing of urine around catheter. Also, urethral stricture formation, meatal tears, encrustation and bladder calculi, urethral perforation, pain, bleeding, bladder spasm, reduced bladder capacity, catheter blockage, latex sensitivity, altered body image, difficulties with sexual relations.

5 Within 48 hours of prostate surgery; history of urethral stricture; history of bacteraemia associated with catheterisation unless patient has been given appropriate prophylaxis (discuss with microbiologist); priapism (a persistent and usually painful erection of the penis that requires urgent decompression).

6 Catheter valve: every 7 days; catheter drainage bags: 7 days; catheter 'belly bags': every 28 days.

7 Talcum powder and creams must not be used around catheter sites.

8 Catheter type, length and size; batch number; manufacturer; amount of water instilled into the balloon; date and time of catheterisation; reasons for catheterisation; colour of urine drained; any problems negotiated during the procedure; a review date to assess the need for continued catheterisation, or date of change of catheter.

9 From the sample port on the drainage bag. The port must be cleaned prior to the procedure. Urine samples must never be taken by emptying the bag via the drainage tap.

10 After emptying catheter bag the port should be decontaminated with alcohol wipes.

CHAPTER 6

Activity 6.1

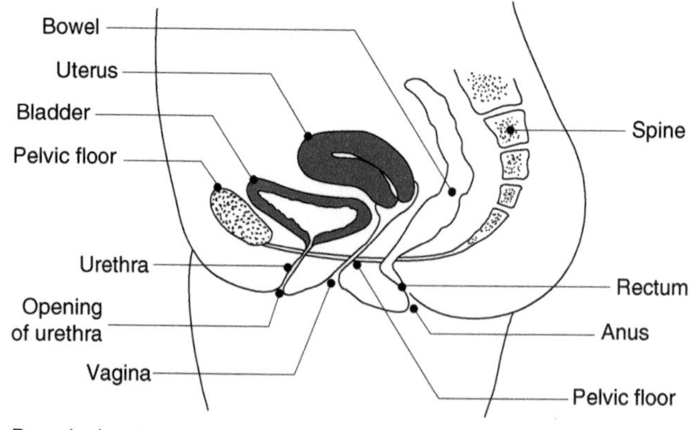

Permission to reproduce this image is granted by North Bristol NHS Trust and University Hospitals Bristol NHS Foundation Trust

Questions

6.1 If you take out the catheter tube, subsequent tubes may follow the same tract into the vagina. By leaving the tube in place, we will hopefully avoid this wrong tract a second time.

Test Your Knowledge

1. Gain consent.
2. From the pubic bone at the front to the bottom of the backbone.
3. Soap and water.
4. For the same reasons as male catheterisation: for drainage, investigation and instillation purposes. It may also be performed during childbirth.
5. PureWick.
6. No, males also have pelvic floors.

CHAPTER 7

Activity 7.1

Lettuce = 0.5 g + cucumber = 0.5 g + tomato = 1 g + coleslaw = 1 g + baked potato = 5.0 g + potato salad = 1.6 g + slice of white bread = 1.0 g = 10.6 g in total.

Questions

7.1 (i) Storage: the colon stores unabsorbed food residue. Within 72 hours of intake, 70% of food residue has been excreted. The remaining 30% stays in the colon for up to a week. The longer food residue remains in the colon, the more water is absorbed and the harder the stools that are produced. (ii) Absorption: sodium, water, chloride and some fat-soluble vitamins are all absorbed from the colon. Some drugs, for example some steroids and aspirin, are also absorbed by the colon. (iii) Secretion: mucus is secreted by the colon to lubricate the faeces and aid expulsion. (iv) Synthesis of some vitamins: bacteria which colonise the colon are responsible for the production of small amounts of vitamin K, thiamine, folic acid and riboflavin. (v) Elimination: the main function of the colon is the absorption of fluid and the peristaltic movement of faecal matter into the rectum, which has sensory nerve endings that generate the sensation of fullness, followed by a desire to defecate.

7.2 Impaction with faecal overflow, pelvic floor damage, neurological disease (such as cerebral disease, spinal cord problems), colon disorders (such as carcinoma, colitis, diverticulitis, irritable bowel syndrome), surgical trauma, diarrhoea (caused by infections such as gastroenteritis), endocrine disorders (such as diabetes).

Test Your Knowledge

1. Storage, absorption, secretion, synthesis of some vitamins, elimination.
2. The Bristol Stool Chart.
3. Digital rectal examination.
4. Autonomic dysreflexia.
5. Distended bladder (e.g. catheter blockage or bladder outlet obstruction), distended bowel (e.g. constipation or impaction or full rectum), ingrown toenail, fracture

below level of the lesion, pressure ulcer, contact burn, scald or sunburn, urinary tract infections or bladder spasms, renal or bladder calculi, pain or trauma, deep vein thrombosis, over-stimulation during sexual activity, severe anxiety.

6 To trigger reflex relaxation of internal sphincter and promote emptying of the rectum.

7 Haemorrhoids, anal fissures, faecal impaction, rectal prolapse.

8 15 g.

9 30 g.

10 Yes.

CHAPTER 8

Questions

8.1 Ileal conduit: this is where the ureters are diverted from the bladder into a new 'bladder sac', usually part of the bowel; the new ileal conduit. The other end of the ileal conduit opens on to the surface of the skin: the stoma.
Nephrostomy: this is where a long tube is placed straight into the kidney. At the other end of tube, a collection bag is attached for urine drainage.

8.2 Large bowel diversion = colostomy; small bowel diversion = ileostomy; urinary diversion = urostomy, ileal conduit or nephrostomy

Test Your Knowledge

1 Urostomy, ileal conduit or nephrostomy.

2 The area of skin around the stoma site.

3 Irritable bowel syndrome (bowel), ulcerated colitis (bowel), cancer (bowel or urinary), diverticulitis or Crohn's disease (bowel), trauma (bowel or urinary), neurological damage (urinary or bowel), cancer of the pelvis (urinary or bowel), congenital disorder (urinary or bowel).

4 The drainage bag may not stick to the skin if certain commercial preparations are used.

5 False – biodegradable bags can be flushed.

6 False – there is no sensation in the stoma.

7 False – an ileostomy is formed from the small intestine.

8 False – a colostomy is formed from the large intestine.

9 False – this digestive bacteria is called *Escherichia coli*.

10 True – faeces in the ileostomy are more liquid.

CHAPTER 9

Test Your Knowledge

1 Tenacious: holding or sticking firmly. In other words, thick sticky secretions. Would be treated with nebulisation to thin the secretions to make them easier to remove by suction.

Bifurcating: a point at which division of two branches occurs, such as in the bronchial tree descending into the lungs.

Kyphoscoliosis: kyphosis combined with scoliosis. Abnormal curvature of the spine both forwards and sideways.

INR: international normalised ratio – a measurement of blood clotting time. The higher the INR, the longer it will take for your blood to clot.

2 8–10 G.

3 20–25 mmHg.

4 Softening of the skin around the stoma site (known as the peristomal skin).

5 Yes.

CHAPTER 10

Activity 10.1

1 pH 4.5–8.0.

2 Diabetic ketoacidosis, starvation, potassium depletion, high-protein diet.

3 The formation of renal calculi (stones).

4 Urinary tract infection, excessive vomiting, consumption of large amounts of antacids, diet high in vegetables, citrus fruits and dairy products.

5 A stale urine specimen.

Test Your Knowledge

1 Urine pH, protein, glucose, ketones and blood.

2 Two hours

3 Away from flammable substances and potential ignition sources.

4 The upper outer aspects of the fingers or the outer heel for babies.

5 Low blood sugar level.

6 Vegetarians often have a pH that is above 9.

CHAPTER 11

Questions

11.1 (i) Obtaining blood to rule out medical conditions, such as obtaining electrolyte levels (e.g. sodium, potassium and urea). (ii) To monitor levels of blood components, such as obtaining a full blood count to ascertain the number of red blood cells and their quality. (iii) Obtaining a crossmatch prior to surgery. (iv) Obtaining blood for diagnosis, such as cardiac enzymes, and liver function (e.g. enzymes released by the liver) and blood glucose readings. (iv) To monitor blood levels, such as looking at levels of drugs in the blood, such as warfarin and phenytoin, which can be toxic.

11.2 Full blood count, ESR, CRP, LFT, U's and E's, aPTT, PT, INR, Calcium, Cholesterol, Glucose, D-Dimer, Troponin.

Test Your Knowledge

1 It is recommended that a tourniquet should not be left in place for more than one minute; this also promotes patient comfort.

2 It has been shown to alter some blood results.

3 The blood sample tubes must be taken in that order, as recommended by the manufacturer or pathology laboratory.

4 Adults over 18 years are presumed able to give consent (with mental capacity).
5 Hepatitis B.
6 Valid consent.
7 The time at which the last dose of the drug was taken.
8 A differential blood count identifies the concentrations of white blood cells in the blood.
9 Neutrophils, lymphocytes, monocytes, eosinophils and basophils.
10 Clotting studies, international normalised ratio, heparin monitoring, warfarin monitoring, D-Dimer.

CHAPTER 12

Questions

12.1 (i) Fluid and electrolyte replacement; (ii) intravenous drug therapy; (iii) transfusions; (iv) prophylaxis; (v) the administration of dyes and contrast media.

12.2 Extravasation – when a vesicant (blister-forming) substance eats away at the underlying tissue due to a cannula coming out of a vein. Infiltration occurs when a cannula dislodges from a vein and the infused substance enters the surrounding tissues. The area can become oedematous (very swollen). It used to be referred to as 'tissuing'.

Test Your Knowledge

1 Usually only immediately after the cannula has first been inserted.
2 The push–pause technique.
3 Always use the smallest possible cannula in the largest possible vein.
4 1.9 litres per hour.
5 Nothing smaller than a 10-ml syringe, otherwise, too much pressure may be applied.
6 Visual inspection of phlebitis.
7 Povidone iodine 10%.
8 Caused by rubbing and irritating the lining of the vein (tunica intima).

CHAPTER 13

Activity 13.1

We use the following formula, remembering that clear fluids are administered at 20 drops per ml:

$$\text{rate} = \frac{\text{volume}}{\text{time in hours}} \times \text{drops per millilitre} / 60 \text{ minutes}$$

So:

$$\frac{1000 \text{ ml}}{8 \text{ hours}} \times \frac{20 \text{ drops per ml}}{60 \text{ minutes}} = 42 \text{ drops per minute.}$$

Now we need to adjust the drip rate to get this medication back on track, using three steps.

1 How much of the bag is left?
2 How much time is left?
3 Use the formula:

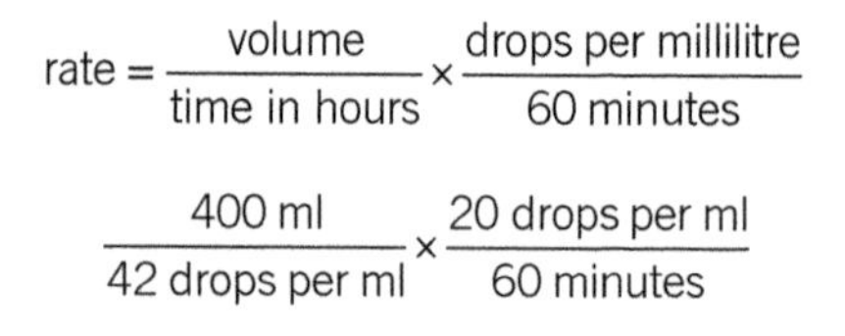

$$\text{rate} = \frac{\text{volume}}{\text{time in hours}} \times \frac{\text{drops per millilitre}}{60 \text{ minutes}}$$

$$\frac{400 \text{ ml}}{42 \text{ drops per ml}} \times \frac{20 \text{ drops per ml}}{60 \text{ minutes}}$$

= 3.17 drops per minute.

So, we change the drip rate to approximately three drops per minute.

We would need to inform the patient that a drug error has occurred and complete all documentation in relation to this. A doctor will also need to be informed.

Activity 13.2

This drug should be given as follows:

$$\frac{\text{dose}}{\text{rate}} = \frac{20 \text{ mg}}{4 \text{ mg per minute}}$$
$$= \text{give over 5 minutes}$$

Activity 13.3

- As a nursing associate who has not yet been competency assessed intravenous administration, you will need to work under supervision until you have been assessed., but as you have attended the study day, you can be a 'second checker'.
- Handwashing is an infection control measure that a nurse must undertake before and after a drug administration.
- Wearing gloves during drug preparation may not be in your own medicine management policy or that of the Royal Marsden. However, anecdotally nurses have reported experiencing problems such as resistance to antibiotics because they have not worn gloves in the past during the procedure; it is therefore considered best practice to wear gloves during the preparation.
- Poor infection control measure by sitting on patient's bed and use of a pulp tray (cardboard); should be using a plastic rigid tray and an integral sharps bin.
- Drugs should not be left unattended and on patient's bed, particularly if sharps are present.
- All peripheral cannulas should be assessed prior to use for signs of phlebitis and to ensure that the device is in working order.
- Poor and unsafe practice leading to needle-stick injury – sharps bin should only be three quarters full and the practitioner should not force any sharp device into a sharps bin.

Questions

13.1 (1)Foods; (2)injected venom; (3)drugs; (4)latex.

13.2 Cephalosporin antibiotics: a group of semi-synthetic antibiotics derived from the mould *Cephalosporium*. Used to treat a variety of infections. Sulfa antibiotics are derived from sulfanilamide, which prevents the growth of bacteria. Allopurinol: a drug used in the treatment of gout by reducing the level of uric acid in the blood and tissues.

13.3 No. Patients with anaphylaxis can deteriorate if made to sit up or stand up. Lie the patient down and raise their feet.

Test Your Knowledge

1 The mistakes are:
   - Flagyl is a trade name and should have been prescribed as metronidazole.

- Intravenous metronidazole should be prescribed every eight hours, which is TDS (three times a day) and not QDS (four times a day). The patient has been given the drug four times in one day instead of three times in 24 hours.
- Cefuroxime is prescribed as QDS: this is correct as this drug can be prescribed QDS or TDS; that is, every six or eight hours.
- These two antibiotics can be mixed, but TDS drugs are usually given at 08:00, 16:00 and 24:00 and QDS drugs are usually given at 06:00, 12:00, 18:00 and 24:00; we can see only once in 24 hours can these drugs actually be given together. It is also not a good idea to mix antibiotics because if the patient has a reaction we will not know which drug has caused the reaction.
- Adverse effects of metronidazole include gastrointestinal disturbances, such as nausea and vomiting: is our patient having a reaction to the medications, or an overdose of medication?
- Did anyone check whether Mrs Jones is allergic to antibiotics by asking her or checking her notes? Are we seeing the start of an anaphylaxis event?
- Just because the registered nurse was a very experienced nurse, did the student not check all prescriptions herself? Why not?
- A student nurse without a PIN number (that's a nurse's unique identification number, issued by the Nursing and Midwifery Council) should not be a second checker. Student nurses can be a third checker only, because they have not yet been assessed for the administration of intravenous medications.
- Documentation should be completed following the drug error, but first the patient should be told of the error and apologies given.
- A doctor would need to be informed of the drug error.
- The patient would require close observation.

2 This is a classic case of phlebitis and is not a usual reaction to intravenous therapy. You will need to remove the cannula at once and inform the doctor immediately. The service user will need to be reassured and all your actions should be documented and reported.

3 Children = food.

4 Adult = drugs.

5 During anaphylaxis, the blood vessels leak, bronchial tissues swell and the blood pressure drops, causing choking and collapse. Adrenalin acts to constrict blood vessels, relax the smooth muscles in the lungs, stimulates heart contractility and help stop swelling around the face and lips (angio-oedema).

6 Food triggers include peanuts, tree nuts (walnuts, pecans, pistachios, cob nuts, cashews, almonds), shellfish, fish, milk, pulses (lentils), sesame, soy, wheat, eggs, some fruit and vegetables.

CHAPTER 14

Activity 14.1

Washed cells: here, the plasma proteins are washed away from the plasma, leaving the cells only. This procedure is performed on blood for individuals who have previously reacted to a transfusion. This procedure is very expensive and is performed by the National Blood Transfusion Service.

CMV stands for cytomegalovirus, a type of herpes virus related to the cold sore, which many of us carry. In people with strong immune systems the virus remains inactive, but those with compromised immune systems need to have their transfused blood more finely filtered to remove any traces of the virus.

Irradiated blood is given to patients with conditions such as Hodgkin's disease and for babies in utero.

Activity 14.2

- Registered or student nurse/midwife, nursing associate, assistant practitioner and trainee assistant practitioner.
- Operating department practitioner/assistant.
- Healthcare assistant.
- Ward clerk/receptionist.
- Designated theatre porters.

But only if trained to do so.

Activity 14.3

Red blood cells are stored in the fridge at 2–6°C. They must be returned to the fridge and signed back in after 30 minutes if not going to be put up immediately. Platelets and fresh frozen plasma (FFP) will not be stored in the fridge, but can be obtained from the laboratory. This is because platelets need to be kept moving as they want to do what comes naturally, which is clumping together to create a fibrin mesh. Clot formation is a safety measure to stop us from bleeding to death every time we have a cut. FFP is frozen to minus 30°C and needs to be thawed by the laboratory and then transfused immediately.

Test Your Knowledge

1. Temperature, pulse, blood pressure and respiratory rate; these need to be done before collection, 15 minutes after transfusion starts and at the end of transfusion.
2. Temperature rises by one degree C.
3. 2.1 million.
4. NHS Blood and Transport, Northern Ireland, Scottish National Blood Transfusion Service, Welsh Blood Services.
5. Cryoprecipitate.
6. IBCT = incorrect blood component transfused.

CHAPTER 15

Activity 15.1

U = Uniform.

Test Your Knowledge

1. 30 : 2.
2. 5–6 cm depth.
3. 15 : 2, but starting with five rescue breaths.

4 4 cm.
5 100 compressions per minute (not greater than 120 per minute).
6 100 compressions per minute (not greater than 120 per minute).
7 Kilo.
8 Automated external defibrillator.
9 Recommended summary plan for emergency care and treatment.
10 W – whiskey (or whisky – does not matter if spelt the Scottish or Irish way!).

CHAPTER 16

Questions

16.1 A standard electrocardiogram machine has 10 leads to attach to 10 electrodes on the body, which actually produces 12 electrical views of the heart.

16.2 The patient does not need to lie down flat; many patients are unable to tolerate this. Supine position is best with knees flexed as this reduces the cardiac labour of heart muscle if patient has chest pain.

Test Your Knowledge

1 b.
2 d.
3 a and b.
4 c.
5 False: the T wave shows as a negative on someone experiencing a myocardial infarction.
6 False: a normal electrocardiogram should show sinus rhythm.

Appendix 1

NEWS 2 OBSERVATION CHART

NEWS key: 0 1 2 3	FULL NAME	
	DATE OF BIRTH	DATE OF ADMISSION

Parameter	Range	Score	Range
	DATE		DATE
	TIME		TIME
A+B Respirations Breaths/min	≥25	3	≥25
	21–24	2	21–24
	18–20		18–20
	15–17		15–17
	12–14		12–14
	9–11	1	9–11
	≤8	3	≤8
A+B SpO_2 Scale 1 Oxygen saturation (%)	≥96		≥96
	94–95	1	94–95
	92–93	2	92–93
	≤91	3	≤91
SpO_2 Scale 2[†] Oxygen saturation (%) Use Scale 2 if target range is 88–92%, eg in hypercapnic respiratory failure	≥97 on O_2	3	≥97 on O_2
	95–96 on O_2	2	95–96 on O_2
	93–94 on O_2	1	93–94 on O_2
	≥93 on air		≥93 on air
	88–92		88–92
	86–87	1	86–87
[†]ONLY use Scale 2 under the direction of a qualified clinician	84–85	2	84–85
	≤83%	3	≤83%
Air or oxygen?	A=Air		A=Air
	O_2 L/min	2	O_2 L/min
	Device		Device
C Blood pressure mmHg Score uses systolic BP only	≥220	3	≥220
	201–219		201–219
	181–200		181–200
	161–180		161–180
	141–160		141–160
	121–140		121–140
	111–120		111–120
	101–110	1	101–110
	91–100	2	91–100
	81–90	3	81–90
	71–80	3	71–80
	61–70	3	61–70
	51–60	3	51–60
	≤50	3	≤50
C Pulse Beats/min	≥131	3	≥131
	121–130	2	121–130
	111–120	2	111–120
	101–110	1	101–110
	91–100	1	91–100
	81–90		81–90
	71–80		71–80
	61–70		61–70
	51–60		51–60
	41–50	1	41–50
	31–40	3	31–40
	≤30	3	≤30
D Consciousness Score for NEW onset of confusion (no score if chronic)	Alert		Alert
	Confusion	3	Confusion
	V	3	V
	P	3	P
	U	3	U
E Temperature °C	≥39.1°	2	≥39.1°
	38.1–39.0°	1	38.1–39.0°
	37.1–38.0°		37.1–38.0°
	36.1–37.0°		36.1–37.0°
	35.1–36.0°	1	35.1–36.0°
	≤35.0°	3	≤35.0°
NEWS TOTAL			TOTAL
	Monitoring frequency		Monitoring
	Escalation of care Y/N		Escalation
	Initials		Initials

Index

Clinical Skills for Nurses, Second Edition. Claire Boyd.